Trichotillomania, Skin Picking, and Other Body-Focused Repetitive Behaviors

Trichotillomania, Skin Picking, and Other Body-Focused Repetitive Behaviors

Edited by

Jon E. Grant, M.D., M.P.H., J.D.
Dan J. Stein, M.D., Ph.D.
Douglas W. Woods, Ph.D.
Nancy J. Keuthen, Ph.D.

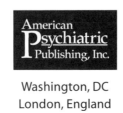

American Psychiatric Publishing, Inc.

Washington, DC
London, England

Copyright © 2012 American Psychiatric Association
ALL RIGHTS RESERVED

Manufactured in the United States of America on acid-free paper
15 14 13 12 11   5 4 3 2 1
First Edition

Typeset in Adobe's Janson and Myriad.

American Psychiatric Publishing, Inc.
1000 Wilson Boulevard
Arlington, VA 22209-3901
www.appi.org

Library of Congress Cataloging-in-Publication Data
Trichotillomania, skin picking, and other body-focused repetitive behaviors / edited by Jon E. Grant ... [et al.]. — 1st ed.
    p. ; cm.
    Includes bibliographical references and index.
    ISBN 978-1-58562-398-3 (pbk. : alk. paper)
1. Compulsive hair pulling. 2. Cognitive therapy. 3. Self-injurious behavior.
I. Grant, Jon E. II. American Psychiatric Publishing.
    [DNLM: 1. Trichotillomania—diagnosis. 2. Cognitive Therapy. 3. Self-Injurious Behavior. 4. Stereotypic Movement Disorder—diagnosis. WM 190]
    RC569.5.H34T76 2012
    616.85'84—dc22
                                                                                    2011010604

British Library Cataloguing in Publication Data
A CIP record is available from the British Library.

CONTENTS

Part 1

CLINICAL CHARACTERISTICS

Part 2

DIAGNOSIS AND EVALUATION

Part 3

TREATMENT

CONTRIBUTORS

Diana Antinoro, Psy.D.
Clinical Director, Child and Adolescent OCD, Tic, Trich, and Anxiety Study Group (COTTAGe), Department of Psychiatry, University of Pennsylvania School of Medicine, Philadelphia, Pennsylvania

Kristin Benavides, B.A.
Research Coordinator, Child and Adolescent OCD, Tic, Trich, and Anxiety Study Group (COTTAGe), Department of Psychiatry, University of Pennsylvania School of Medicine, Philadelphia, Pennsylvania

Samuel R. Chamberlain, M.D., Ph.D.
Department of Psychiatry, University of Cambridge, Addenbrooke's Hospital, Cambridge; National Treatment Service for OCD (England), Hertfordshire Partnership NHS Foundation Trust, Queen Elizabeth II Hospital, Welwyn Garden City, Hertfordshire, United Kingdom

Flint M. Espil, M.A.
University of Wisconsin–Milwaukee, Milwaukee, Wisconsin

Naomi A. Fineberg, M.B.B.S., M.R.C.Psych.
Consultant Psychiatrist, Department of Psychiatry, University of Cambridge, Addenbrooke's Hospital, Cambridge; National Treatment Service for OCD (England), Hertfordshire Partnership NHS Foundation Trust, Queen Elizabeth II Hospital, Welwyn Garden City, Hertfordshire; Postgraduate School of Medicine, University of Hertfordshire, College Lane, Hatfield, United Kingdom

Christopher A. Flessner, Ph.D.
Research Fellow in Psychiatry (Clinical Psychology), Department of Psychiatry and Human Behavior, Bradley Hasbro Children's Research Center, Brown Medical School, Providence, Rhode Island

Martin E. Franklin, Ph.D.
Associate Professor of Clinical Psychology in Psychiatry, University of Pennsylvania School of Medicine; Director, Child and Adolescent OCD, Tic, Trich & Anxiety Group (COTTAGe), Department of Psychiatry, University of Pennsylvania School of Medicine, Philadelphia, Pennsylvania

Patrick C. Friman, Ph.D., ABPP
Boys Town, Nebraska

Mayumi Okada Gianoli
Washington University, St. Louis, Missouri

Ruth G. Golomb, M.Ed., LCPC
Behavior Therapy Center of Greater Washington, Silver Spring, Maryland

Jon E. Grant, M.D., M.P.H., J.D.
Professor, Department of Psychiatry, University of Minnesota, Minneapolis, Minnesota

Nancy J. Keuthen, Ph.D.
Associate Professor of Psychology (Psychiatry), Harvard Medical School; Co-Director, Trichotillomania Clinic and Research Unit; and Chief Psychologist, Obsessive Compulsive Disorder Clinic and Research Unit, Massachusetts General Hospital, Boston, Massachusetts

Christine Lochner, Ph.D.
Associate Professor, Department of Psychiatry, Stellenbosch University, Tygerberg, South Africa

Charles S. Mansueto, Ph.D.
Behavior Therapy Center of Greater Washington, Silver Spring, Maryland

Ladan Mostaghimi, M.D.
Director, Psychocutaneous Medicine Clinic, Department of Dermatology, University of Wisconsin, Madison, Wisconsin

Suzanne Mouton-Odum, Ph.D.
Private Practice

Brian L. Odlaug, B.A.
Graduate Student, Ambulatory Research Center, Department of Psychiatry, University of Minnesota, Minneapolis, Minnesota

Hannah Reese, Ph.D.
Massachusetts General Hospital and Harvard Medical School, Boston, Massachusetts

Kate E. Rogers, B.A.
Behavior Therapy Center of Greater Washington, Silver Spring, Maryland

Jedidiah Siev, Ph.D.
Massachusetts General Hospital and Harvard Medical School, Boston, Massachusetts

Ivar Snorrason, M.A.
University of Wisconsin–Milwaukee, Milwaukee, Wisconsin

Greg Snyder, Ph.D.
Boys Town, Nebraska

Dan J. Stein, M.D., Ph.D.
Professor, Department of Psychiatry and Mental Health, University of Cape Town, Cape Town, South Africa

David F. Tolin, Ph.D., ABPP
Founder and Director, The Institute of Living, Hartford, Connecticut; Adjunct Associate Professor of Psychiatry, Yale University School of Medicine, New Haven, Connecticut

Douglas W. Woods, Ph.D.
Professor, Department of Psychology, University of Wisconsin–Milwaukee, Milwaukee, Wisconsin

DISCLOSURE OF COMPETING INTERESTS

The following contributors to this book have indicated a financial interest in or other affiliation with a commercial supporter, a manufacturer of a commercial product, a provider of a commercial service, a nongovernmental organization, and/ or a government agency, as listed below:

Jon E. Grant, M.D., M.P.H., J.D.—Dr. Grant's research is supported by a grant from the National Institute on Drug Abuse (RC1-DA028279-01) and a Center for Excellence in Gambling Research grant from the Institute for Responsible Gaming. Dr. Grant has received research grants from Psyadon Pharmaceuticals and the University of South Florida, and research support from Forest Pharmaceuticals for investigator-initiated study.

Brian L. Odlaug, B.A.—Mr. Odlaug has received honoraria from Oxford University Press and Current Medicine Group, L.L.C.

Dan J. Stein, M.D., Ph.D.—Dr. Stein has received research grants and/or consultancy honoraria from AstraZeneca, Eli Lilly, GlaxoSmithKline, Johnson & Johnson, Lundbeck, Orion, Pfizer, Pharmacia, Roche, Servier, Solvay, Sumitomo, Tikvah, and Wyeth.

David F. Tolin, Ph.D., ABPP—Dr. Tolin has received research support from Endo Pharmaceuticals, Organon/Schering-Plough, and Pfizer, and royalties from Oxford University Press and Springer.

Douglas W. Woods, Ph.D.—Dr. Woods reports receiving royalties from Oxford University Press, Guilford Press, New Harbinger, and Springer Publications. He also reports receiving honoraria for CME presentations from the Tourette Syndrome Association.

The following contributors to this book do not have any conflicts of interest to disclose:

Diana Antinoro, Psy.D.
Kristin Benavides, B.A.
Samuel R. Chamberlain, M.D., Ph.D.
Flint M. Espil, M.A.
Naomi A. Fineberg, M.B.B.S., M.R.C.Psych.
Christopher A. Flessner, Ph.D.
Martin E. Franklin, Ph.D.
Patrick C. Friman, Ph.D., ABPP
Mayumi Okada Gianoli
Ruth G. Golomb, M.Ed., LCPC
Nancy J. Keuthen, Ph.D.
Christine Lochner, Ph.D.
Charles S. Mansueto, Ph.D.
Ladan Mostaghimi, M.D.
Suzanne Mouton-Odum, Ph.D.
Hannah Reese, Ph.D.
Kate E. Rogers, B.A.
Jedidiah Siev, Ph.D.
Ivar Snorrason, M.A.
Greg Snyder, Ph.D.

INTRODUCTION

Over the past 10 years, the volume of research on chronic hair pulling (trichotillomania), skin picking, and other body-focused repetitive behaviors (BFRBs; stereotypic movement disorders) has grown significantly. Clinicians throughout the world encounter individuals with these disorders but often have no clear understanding of why someone engages in these behaviors or how to help that person. Patients who struggle with these disorders, as well as their families, are also at a loss as to why these behaviors cannot be more easily controlled. This book provides the latest knowledge about trichotillomania, skin picking, and other BFRBs; discusses how to evaluate individuals with these behaviors; and offers treatment options for readers in an easily accessible format. This cutting-edge, concise, and practical information should be useful for clinicians, researchers, family members, and individuals with these disorders.

The 13 chapters of this book are grouped into three parts, focusing on the clinical presentation of these behaviors, the assessment of these behaviors across the developmental spectrum, and various treatment approaches. The first three chapters (Chapter 1, "Trichotillomania: Epidemiology and Clinical Characteristics"; Chapter 2, "Pathological Skin Picking"; and Chapter 3, "Habitual Stereotypic Movements: A Descriptive Analysis of Four Common Types") highlight the important clinical characteristics of trichotillomania, skin picking, and other BFRBs. Chapter 4 ("Psychobiology of Hair-Pulling Disorder [Trichotillomania] and Skin-Picking Disorder") describes the biological and psychological underpinnings of these behaviors.

A primary aim of this book is to educate clinicians about BFRBs. The second part of this text therefore addresses the diagnosis and evaluation of individuals with these behaviors. Many people engage in these behaviors to some extent; therefore, understanding when a behavior rises to the level of a disorder is important. Chapter 5 ("Diagnosis and Comorbidity") addresses this issue and highlights common co-occurring disorders in these individuals. Often these behaviors stem from, or result in, a variety of skin and hair conditions. Chapter 6 ("Dermatological Assessment of Hair Pulling, Skin Picking, and Nail Biting") provides a thorough dermatological approach to these patients. Trichotillomania and skin picking may manifest differently in different age groups, and Chapter 7 ("Diagnosis and Evaluation: Trichotillomania, Skin Picking, and Other Stereotypic Behaviors in Children") provides an assessment of these behaviors in children and adolescents. Finally, this part concludes with Chapter 8 ("Assessment of Trichotillomania, Pathological Skin Picking, and Stereotypic Movement Disorder"), which discusses the variety of assessment instruments available to clinicians and researchers for more accurate assessment and to record changes in the behaviors over time.

When individuals present with trichotillomania, skin picking, or other BFRBs, clinicians often assume that one size fits all in terms of treatment. Because treatment for these behaviors is complex and requires a deep understanding of the literature, the third part includes chapters on cognitive-behavioral therapy for children and adolescents (Chapter 9, "Cognitive-Behavioral Therapy for Pediatric Trichotillomania") and for adults (Chapter 10, "Cognitive-Behavioral Therapy in Adults"). The last three chapters in this part of the book (Chapter 11, "Alternative Treatments"; Chapter 12, "Pharmacotherapy"; and Chapter 13, "Family Involvement in the Treatment of Children With Body-Focused Repetitive Behaviors") cover other treatment options.

Another aim of this volume is to persuade readers that work on chronic hair pulling, skin picking, and other BFRBs is extremely important. Each of the chapters addresses this theme in one way or another. Many of the chapters, for example, emphasize the enormous distress associated with these conditions as well as their significant morbidity. Although these conditions may not seem to constitute a major public health problem at first blush, on closer examination they appear to represent a key aspect of human suffering. Other chapters highlight the ways in which these conditions provide unique insights into compulsive and impulsive behavior, the reward and stress response systems, and particular aspects of modern pharmacotherapy and psychotherapy. Although these conditions may, at first glance, not seem to be at the forefront of current brain-behavior science, again, a more detailed investigation shows that work on these conditions can intersect with the cutting edge of contemporary research.

In summary, trichotillomania, skin picking, and other BFRBs represent an important and yet largely neglected area of clinical care. As the authors of the chapters in this volume eloquently attest, extraordinary progress has been made in terms of understanding the clinical presentation and diagnosis of these disorders as well as learning how to treat them. Despite this progress, many clinicians who encounter these behaviors do not diagnose them and are not aware of the treatment options for these disorders. Many clinicians are also unaware of the personal and social consequences of these disorders. We hope that clinicians who wish to make more informed decisions regarding the well-being of those who struggle with these disorders will find this text valuable.

Jon E. Grant, M.D., M.P.H., J.D.
Dan J. Stein, M.D., Ph.D.
Douglas W. Woods, Ph.D.
Nancy J. Keuthen, Ph.D.

Part 1

CLINICAL CHARACTERISTICS

Chapter 1

TRICHOTILLOMANIA

Epidemiology and Clinical Characteristics

Charles S. Mansueto, Ph.D.
Kate E. Rogers, B.A.

Trichotillomania is a disorder that may be aptly described as having a long past but a short history. Medical concern with hair pulling has been traced back as far as Hippocrates (Christenson and Mansueto 1999), yet only since 1990 has trichotillomania become the focus of substantial and increased interest by researchers and clinicians. Accordingly, there has been an encouraging growth in our understanding of the nature, course, and clinical features of the disorder. There is increasing awareness of the impact of trichotillomania in terms of the number of sufferers as well as the degree of personal distress associated with the disorder. Although many unanswered questions remain, a richer and more detailed picture of trichotillomania can now be drawn. In this chapter, we describe the current state of our knowledge and understanding with regard to the epidemiology and clinical characteristics of trichotillomania.

EPIDEMIOLOGY

Prevalence

Trichotillomania was once considered a rare disorder, with a reported prevalence rate of only 0.05% (Schachter 1961). Today, however, it is recognized as being much more common than previously believed, with reported rates as high as 4.4% (Grant et al. 2005). Over the years, a wide range of prevalence rates has been reported in the literature, due in part to inconsistencies in the application of diagnostic criteria. In general, rates increase when less stringent diagnostic criteria are applied. Table 1–1 presents the DSM-IV-TR diagnostic criteria for trichotillomania (American Psychiatric Association 2000).

Christenson et al. (1991b) surveyed 2,579 undergraduate students across multiple college campuses and found that 0.6% of these students met full diagnostic criteria for trichotillomania at some point in their lives. Stanley et al. (1994) surveyed 288 college students and found hair pulling in 15.3% of this sample. Grant et al. (2005), in a study of the prevalence of impulse-control disorders in 204 psychiatric inpatients, found a prevalence rate of 3.4% for current trichotillomania among this population, compared with a lifetime prevalence rate of 4.4%.

More recently, Duke et al. (2009) assessed the prevalence of trichotillomania among 830 adults. Although they found that only 0.6% of their total sample met full diagnostic criteria, 6.51% of the total sample reported hair pulling unrelated to grooming activities. Perhaps the most significant finding in this study was that 1.2% of the total sample experienced "clinically significant" hair pulling. Despite the progressive recognition of trichotillomania as substantially more common than once believed, some researchers maintain that its prevalence remains underestimated (Duke et al. 2009).

Discrepancies between reported prevalence rates of trichotillomania are glaring, and although epidemiological data are growing, significant limitations remain. These limitations include small sample sizes, transient symptoms, subthreshold symptoms, and widespread disagreements about operational definitions and diagnostic criteria.

Prevalence Rates Among African Americans

An increasing amount of interest has emerged regarding the prevalence of trichotillomania in the African American community. In 2002, McCarley et al. studied the prevalence of hair pulling in 176 African American and 422 non–African American undergraduate students. Among this sample, African American women reported the highest rate of hair pulling that resulted in noticeable hair loss. However, no significant difference was found between groups for the prevalence of hair pulling that met full diagnostic criteria for trichotillomania.

In another study, Mansueto et al. (2007) examined hair pulling in 248 African American undergraduate students. Among this sample, 6.3% of participants reported having engaged in hair-pulling behavior. Although 15.4% of these individuals reported pulling to the point of noticeable hair loss, most did not meet full diagnostic criteria for trichotillomania. Perhaps the most interesting finding in this study was that African American pullers did not report significant distress or negative functional impact as a result of their

---

TABLE 1–1.   DSM-IV-TR diagnostic criteria for trichotillomania

---

A. Recurrent pulling out of one's hair resulting in noticeable hair loss.

B. An increasing sense of tension immediately before pulling out the hair or when attempting to resist the behavior.

C. Pleasure, gratification, or relief when pulling out the hair.

D. The disturbance is not better accounted for by another mental disorder and is not due to a general medical condition (e.g., a dermatological condition).

E. The disturbance causes clinically significant distress or impairment in social, occupational, or other important areas of functioning.

Source.   Reprinted from American Psychiatric Association: *Diagnostic and Statistical Manual of Mental Disorders*, 4th Edition, Text Revision. Washington, DC, American Psychiatric Association, 2000. Copyright 2000, American Psychiatric Association. Used with permission.

hair-pulling behavior. This finding may support the existence of elevated levels of resiliency among the African American community, but further research is needed to determine the role of this potential factor.

Prevalence Rates Across Cultures

Hair pulling certainly does not seem to occur exclusively in the United States. In a study of 794 Israeli adolescents, hair pulling was found at a lifetime prevalence rate of 1% (King et al. 1995). In a survey of 118 Polish dermatologists (Szepietowski et al. 2009), 68% reported having observed at least one patient with trichotillomania. Five percent of the dermatologists surveyed reported having seen more than 10 patients with trichotillomania.

Onset

Trichotillomania can arise at any age; however, the average age at onset is approximately 13 years (Christenson et al. 1991b). Interestingly, trichotillomania tends to arise during either early childhood or adolescence (Swedo and Rapoport 1991). This bimodal onset has led researchers to investigate whether there may be discrete phenomenological differences between early- and later-onset trichotillomania. For example, later onset has been associated with increased symptom severity, increased treatment resistance, and increased comorbidity (Keuthen et al. 2001). In contrast, early onset often involves transient symptoms and little need for intervention (Walsh and McDougle 2001; Wright and Holmes 2003).

Course

It is important to note that the course of trichotillomania may vary from individual to individual (Keuthen et al. 1998). Trichotillomania is most often considered to be a chronic disorder that tends to fluctuate over time (Flessner et al. 2009). Flessner et al. (2009), in a study of 1,471 females with trichotillomania, found that although symptom severity remains relatively stable over time, the functional impact of these symptoms may fluctuate. They also compared the course of illness in individuals with automatic pulling and those with focused pulling. Although significant fluctuation was not found in automatic pulling, significant fluctuation was found in focused pulling (corresponding to psychological distress and age-related biological changes, such as puberty).

Sex Differences

In young children, trichotillomania seems to be relatively evenly distributed between sexes (Reeve 1999), although a variety of competing findings exist. It is especially difficult to gain a clear picture of the sex distribution of trichotillomania among children because the existing literature includes only studies with very small samples and wide varieties of age ranges. Among the adult population, the sex distribution is even less definitive. Duke et al. (2009) found no significant difference in prevalence of non–clinically significant hair pulling between males and females, whereas Christenson (1995) found that 92.5% of the adult patients presenting to a trichotillomania clinic were female. The research regarding the sex distribution of trichotillomania in adults is largely muddled by differences found between community and clinical samples. Research using community samples has found a relatively even distribution between males and females. Among clinical samples, however, trichotillomania is found in significantly more females than males (Duke et al. 2010).

A variety of theories have been generated to explain this apparent shift in sex distribution. Men can conceal hair pulling more effectively than women due to the natural occurrence of hair loss among aging men. Christenson et al. (1991a) suggested that this ability to maintain the secrecy of their hair-pulling behavior may simply lead men to present for treatment less often than women. An alternative theory is that the discrepancy between the number of men and the number of women with trichotillomania may be due to hormonal differences. For example, premenstrual symptom exacerbation has been reported for hair pulling, urge intensity, urge frequency, and ability to control hair pulling (Keuthen et al. 1997).

Whether there are differences in the clinical presentation of trichotillomania between sexes has also been discussed. In 1994, Christenson et al. studied the clinical presentation of trichotillomania in 128 females and 14 males.

They found few differences between sexes and concluded that, overall, the phenomenology of the disorder is very similar in males and females. In a similar study, Grant and Christenson (2007) examined the presentation of grooming disorders (i.e., trichotillomania or pathological skin picking) in 77 adults. Although they found more similarities than differences between sexes, they did find that in men there was later onset, greater functional impairment, and higher likelihood of suffering from a comorbid anxiety disorder.

Limitations of Epidemiological Data

It is important to recognize the limitations of the epidemiological data regarding trichotillomania. The literature is still relatively young in its development, which makes the research especially vulnerable to pitfalls such as small sample sizes, transient symptoms, subthreshold symptoms, and variability among diagnostic criteria.

The existing epidemiological data on trichotillomania are fundamentally limited by the use of small sample sizes in relevant empirical studies. Sample size plays a vital role in determining the generalizability of a study's findings, because a large sample size is more representative of the population at large.

The epidemiological picture of trichotillomania is also clouded by the existence of transient symptoms—those symptoms that resolve as spontaneously as they arise. It may be misleading to equate the prevalence rates of transient and chronic trichotillomania. This is a particularly prominent issue with regard to childhood trichotillomania, because transient symptoms most often occur in early childhood (O'Sullivan et al. 1997). Mehregan (1970) reported that the number of children with trichotillomania may be as much as seven times the number of adults with the disorder. This suggests that a large portion of children with trichotillomania experience transient symptoms that resolve prior to adulthood.

Perhaps the most damaging limitation of the epidemiological data is the inconsistent assessment of trichotillomania. Some studies simply measure the occurrence of hair pulling unrelated to grooming activities; some measure the occurrence of hair pulling resulting in noticeable hair loss; some measure the occurrence of "clinically significant" hair pulling; and some measure the occurrence of hair pulling meeting full diagnostic criteria for trichotillomania (see Table 1–2). This use of disparate methods of assessment is especially problematic in the trichotillomania literature because relatively few empirical studies have been conducted. It is important to keep these limitations in mind when considering the validity and implications of the epidemiological data presented regarding trichotillomania.

Although the current state of the epidemiological data is far from perfect, improvements will continue to be made as the limitations just described are

TABLE 1–2.   Prevalence rates by assessment criteria

Assessment criteria	Prevalence, %	Source
Hair pulling unrelated to grooming	15.3	Stanley et al. 1994
	6.5	Duke et al. 2009
Hair pulling + noticeable hair loss	2.0	Rothbaum et al. 1993
	2.5	Christenson et al. 1991b
"Clinically significant" hair pulling	1.2	Duke et al. 2009
Full diagnostic criteria for trichotillomania	0.6	Christenson et al. 1991a
	0.6	Duke et al. 2009

addressed in future research endeavors. Future research should strive to 1) increase sample sizes; 2) consistently apply a standardized assessment of trichotillomania across studies; 3) further investigate the epidemiology of trichotillomania in youths; and 4) conduct longitudinal studies to better understand the course of the disorder and account for transient symptoms. To date, a relatively small number of epidemiological studies of trichotillomania exists, leaving clinicians, researchers, and consumers with limited and conflicting information. In order to progress in our understanding of trichotillomania and how this disorder is represented in the general population, it is vital that the epidemiological literature regarding trichotillomania continues to grow.

CLINICAL CHARACTERISTICS

Although some characteristics of trichotillomania as defined in DSM-IV-TR have been challenged, the hallmark characteristic is clearly the recurrent pulling out of one's own hair. Whereas most early descriptions of trichotillomania in the literature emphasized the mechanistic simplicity of hair pulling, more recent reports have highlighted both the phenomenological complexity and the heterogeneity of the disorder (O'Sullivan et al. 2000).

An early attempt to empirically quantify the phenomenology of trichotillomania, and thereby establish a more complete phenomenological perspective, was reported by Mansueto (1991). He described diverse, idiosyncratic, and heterogeneous subjective and behavioral characteristics of hair pulling in 42 adult female hair-pulling patients. These findings suggested a previously undescribed phenomenological complexity comprising such components as situational variables, motor habits, affective states, cognitive elements, and sensory experiences, each of which played a functional role in repetitive hair-pulling patterns. These included a complex array of behaviors that were beyond the specific act of hair pulling. Later reports essentially corroborated trichotillomania as more phenomenologically complex than previously reported (Christenson et al. 1991a, 1993). Today, trichotillomania is widely regarded as diverse, idiosyncratic, and heterogeneous.

Mansueto et al. (1997) presented a broad conceptual model, the Comprehensive Behavioral (ComB) Model of trichotillomania, that provided a framework for organizing and analyzing the phenomena associated with hair pulling and utilizing these phenomena for research and clinical purposes. The ComB Model provides an organizational framework for the wide array of potentially critical variables associated with trichotillomania in a functional analytic (i.e., an "A-B-C") formulation. This incorporates **A**ntecedents, or cues that generate impulses or urges to pull hair; the complex array of **B**ehaviors involved in the pulling of the hair; and the **C**onsequences of hair pulling that influence its perpetuation. For the remainder of this chapter, phenomenological findings associated with problematic hair pulling are organized and presented within the framework of the ComB Model of trichotillomania.

Antecedent Cues That Foster Hair Pulling

Many, but not all, hair pullers report an impulse or urge to pull that precedes pulling episodes. In such cases, the urges tend to occur within specific circumstances and in response to cues that can precipitate hair pulling. These circumstances and cues can vary greatly both among and within individual hair pullers. In the ComB Model, the variables are divided into two types: 1) *external cues*, such as physical settings in which hair pulling tends to occur (e.g., in the bedroom, at the work desk) and implements that may be employed in hair pulling (e.g., tweezers, magnifying mirrors); and 2) *internal cues*, which comprise cues for pulling that are generated by the individual, including affective (e.g., anxiety), sensory (e.g., itching), and cognitive (e.g., thoughts such as "these gray hairs look awful!") cues.

External Cues

Settings in which hair pulling occurs include the following areas in the home: bedroom, bathroom, living room, family room, and home office. Outside the home, common settings for hair pulling include classrooms, the car, the work desk, and public restrooms (Penzel 2003). The ComB Model suggests that secondary associations may form between external environmental cues and the urge or tendency to pull hair (Mansueto et al. 1997). Implements to aid pulling constitute another category of external cues. Most commonly, wall mirrors, hand mirrors, and tweezers are implements used to facilitate pulling. It is likely that over time, the presence of such implements can serve as cues to precipitate hair-pulling episodes (Mansueto et al. 1997).

Internal Cues

Cues generated within the individual hair puller are characterized by phenomenological richness and complexity. A great deal of attention in the literature has focused on the affective and related factors, such as anger, depression, frustration, indecision, lethargy, fatigue, and embarrassment. "Hurt" feelings were also reported as contributing to episodes of hair pulling in some individuals (Christenson et al. 1993; Mackenzie et al. 1995; Mansueto 1991). Shusterman et al. (2009) offered some corroboration of this view in finding that "boredom seems to be a central, fairly universal affective correlate of hair pulling, followed by anxiety and tension, and then by other emotions" (p. 642). According to the ComB Model, any emotion (even happiness or excitement) can, through associative learning, come to serve as a cue for hair pulling in a given individual (Mansueto et al. 1997).

A second type of internal cue that serves to trigger hair pulling, according to the ComB Model, is sensations, including visual, tactile, and other kinds of bodily sensations. Pruritus (itching) at the site from which hair is pulled apparently serves as a hair-pulling cue in some individuals (Christenson et al. 1991a; Mansueto 1991) and may feature even more prominently among African American hair pullers (Neal-Barnett and Stadulis 2006). Some individuals report diffuse tactile sensations at the pulling site, such as heightened sensitivity, irritation, or pressure, as triggers for hair pulling. Such sensations may also be stimulated by pulling and thus may provide cues for further pulling.

Specific qualities of individual hairs also often provoke pulling in trichotillomania. Hairs that feel coarse, sharp, rough, oily, gritty, or knotted to the touch have been known to cue hair pulling (Mansueto 1991) in some individuals. Because repeated pulling can cause normal hairs to develop textural change, the availability of more "target hairs" can promote increased hair pulling (Christenson 1995). The visual appearance of hairs can also cue pulling in some individuals. For example, gray, split, curly, or dark hairs, as well as hairs judged to be "out of line" or "out of place," can precipitate hair pulling (Mansueto et al. 1997).

Finally, cognitive events such as thoughts and beliefs (e.g., "all the gray hairs must be removed" or "I have to get my eyebrows even") can instigate hair pulling. These can work in conjunction with other triggers (i.e., visual cues and resulting negative feelings) and may represent an interface with qualities of perfectionism or even obsessive-compulsive features (Christenson and Mansueto 1999). Duke et al. (2009) found that the following cognitions were most commonly associated with hair pulling: "feels coarse" (53.3%); "doesn't feel right" (30%); "is curly" (26.7%); and "doesn't look right" (23.3%).

Regarding another aspect of cognition in hair pulling, Christenson et al. (1991a) gave particular emphasis to the role of awareness or lack thereof in trichotillomania. They referred to the degrees to which individuals are aware of their pulling at any given moment as "automatic" versus "focused" pulling. Others had reported that some hair pulling is performed without the individual being fully aware of the activity (Azrin and Nunn 1973; Mansueto 1991) or with the individual even in a trancelike state (Christenson and Mansueto 1999). According to Christenson and Mackenzie (1994), focused pulling occurs when pulling is the center of the person's attention and is accompanied by powerful urges, mounting tension, or thoughts pushing the hair pulling; this is the predominant style in a quarter of trichotillomania patients. Automatic, or unfocused, pulling occurs in the majority of patients at least some of the time that they have pulled hair. Although this was the predominant style for some of the individuals studied by Christenson and Mackenzie, many were focused at least part of the time. Woods et al. (2006) found that a majority of subjects reported being aware of their hair pulling most of the time. Further clarifying the implication of the automatic versus focused dimension, Flessner et al. (2008) found that high-automatic pullers experienced more severe trichotillomania and greater stress than low-automatic pullers. High-focused pullers experienced more severe trichotillomania, greater stress and depression, and greater functional impact than low-focused pullers. An extreme example of automatic pulling was addressed in a report in which 11% of dermatologists surveyed reported that they had seen patients who only pulled hair while sleeping (Murphy et al. 2007). This finding warrants further investigation to rule out the possibility of face-saving untruthfulness by the patients.

Hair-Pulling Behaviors

The term *hair pulling* suggests a simple act—the plucking out of hair. Yet trichotillomania is a complex, highly individualistic disorder, and there is great variation in the manner in which pulling is actually accomplished. The ComB Model identifies a sequence of behaviors that varies from individual to individual. This sequence consists of three stages: 1) preparatory behaviors, 2) pulling behaviors, and 3) disposition activities.

Preparatory Behaviors

Preparatory behaviors consist of actions described previously, such as seeking privacy, acquiring necessary implements, and employing tactile or visual searches for appropriate "target hairs." These behaviors are more character-istic of a focused pulling style, however, and may be largely absent when pull-ing is automatic. Yet touching or stroking of hair usually precedes pulling of either style (Mansueto 1991).

Pulling Behaviors

Generally, hair is pulled with the tips of the thumb and index finger or by twirling the hair around the index finger before pulling. The dominant hand is employed by about half of hair pullers, whereas the nondominant hand is used by about a third of pullers, with approximately a fifth using both domi-nant and nondominant hands (Christenson et al. 1991a). Although hair is sometimes yanked out in tufts, it is usually removed one at a time (Christen-son et al. 1991a; Mansueto 1991).

A number of studies, not surprisingly, have found that the scalp is the most common site for pulling, followed by eyelashes and eyebrows (in de-scending order) (Christenson and Mansueto 1999). Pulling from the pubic area, extremities, and other body locations is less common. Table 1–3 details the hair-pulling practices of 1,697 subjects who participated in a large-scale Internet survey of trichotillomania sufferers (Woods et al. 2006).

The number of hairs removed, the amount of time spent in pulling, the degree of cosmetic damage done, and the patterns and topography of the behavior vary greatly, both among hair pullers and across incidents and time in any given individual. Episodes of pulling can last only moments or up to many hours, with longer ones often described as "binges." Only one, a few, or hundreds of hairs may be removed (Christenson et al. 1991a; Mansueto 1991), sometimes from a particular site and sometimes distributed over larger areas, perhaps in a conscious effort to limit the noticeable damage. Roughly half of individuals with trichotillomania pull hair exclusively from one body site, whereas others pull hair from more than one site (Christenson et al. 1991a; Mansueto 1991).

Disposition Activities

Activities after the pulling of hair are also idiosyncratic and may be complex. Although in some cases pulled hairs are quickly discarded, it is not unusual for individuals to engage in a variety of activities employing the hair or the root—the fleshy bulb that is often attached to the hair shaft. Most hair pullers examine, manipulate, bite, chew, or swallow roots or entire hairs. Some rub hair or roots between their fingertips or on their lips or face; wrap hair around fingers or pull it through their teeth; pull or bite the root off the hair shaft; or save the hair for such uses at a later time (Christenson et al. 1991a; Mansueto 1991). Less common (Grant and Odlaug 2008), but of notable concern, is the

TABLE 1–3. **Hair-pulling practices of 1,697 subjects with trichotillomania in a large-scale Internet survey**

Hair-pulling site	*n*	%
Scalp	1,235	72.8
Brows	957	56.4
Lashes	875	51.6
Pubic area	860	50.7
Legs	370	21.8
Arms	211	12.4
Armpits	210	12.4
Trunk	121	7.1
Mustache	92	5.4
Beard	73	4.3
Other people	7	0.4
Other	122	7.1

Source.   Data derived from the findings of Woods et al. (2006).

eating of whole hairs or parts of hairs in trichotillomania patients. Although nibbling and swallowing small bits of hair or hair roots is probably benign, the ingestion of whole hairs in sufficient quantities can lead to more serious medical complications, including death, when trichobezoars (hair balls) form in the digestive tract (Christenson and Mansueto 1999).

POTENTIALLY REINFORCING CONSEQUENCES OF HAIR PULLING

The ComB Model describes two classes of consequences significant to trichotillomania: *reinforcing consequences* and *aversive consequences.* As with many problems that invoke difficulties with self-control, reinforcing consequences tend to quickly follow the performance of the behavior, whereas aversive consequences tend to occur later. With regard to trichotillomania, many gratifying experiences have the potential to serve as reinforcing events for hair pulling. As mentioned before, tension prior to pulling and relief after pulling are part of the diagnostic criteria for trichotillomania, yet they are clearly not universally found among chronic hair pullers. Some pullers do, however, experience forms of relief or gratification after hair extraction.

Regarding the immediate sensory effects of hair pulling, it seems that the experience of pain plays a relatively small role in adults with trichotillomania (Christenson and Mansueto 1999). Meunier et al. (2009) found that pain was associated with early hair pulling in their pediatric sample but that pleasurable sensations characterized later experiences. It seems clear that distinctly pleasurable feelings are much more likely than pain to result from hair pulling (Christenson and Mansueto 1999), thus providing potentially positively reinforcing consequences for that behavior. The satisfaction derived from the manipulation of hairs or hair roots by handling and oral activities may function similarly to maintain the disorder.

Another type of gratification occurs in trichotillomania when hair pulling functions to eliminate or attenuate aversive sensations and/or negative affective states that exist prior to the removal of hair. Mansueto (1991) reported that some of his subjects experienced relief from unwanted sensations, such as sensitivity, itching, irritation, pressure, and burning sensations localized at the pulling site. Likewise, Woods et al. (2006) found that a high percentage of the above-mentioned, Internet-surveyed hair pullers reported relief from varieties of antecedent somatic phenomena. The ComB Model accommodates these kinds of specific relief as well as elimination or attenuation of less well-defined states associated with hair pulling, such as those typically described as "urges" or "cravings."

The likelihood that hair pulling serves a function of regulating affective states and nervous system arousal has been suggested (Mansueto et al. 1997) and has received increasing attention in recent years (e.g., Penzel 2003). In this view, hair pulling can serve to reduce general tension but can also serve an arousal function to energize individuals out of lethargic states. Mansueto (1991) reported that reduction of boredom was almost equal to tension reduction as a function of hair pulling in his subjects—a finding that was recently corroborated by Shusterman et al. (2009). Diefenbach et al. (2002) interviewed 44 subjects with trichotillomania and found that decreases were reported in boredom, anxiety, and tension immediately after pulling. Penzel (2003) speculated that trichotillomania occurs in individuals whose homeostatic systems are insufficient to regulate arousal and that hair pulling represents an effort to compensate and maintain equilibrium in the nervous system.

Hair pulling may serve a regulation function in a wider range of affective and related states, such as anger, depression, indecision, and fatigue (Mansueto 1991). Shusterman et al. (2009) reported that for subjects who had difficulty regulating a particular emotion, it was *that* emotion that was likely to be experienced before and during hair pulling. In the large-scale, Internet-based survey of 1,697 responders who self-reported symptoms consistent with trichotillomania, individuals with more severe symptoms acknowledged more frequent experiences of physical or mental anxiety prior to pulling and relief, pleasure, or gratification occurring after pulling (Woods et al. 2006). Thus, evidence suggests that hair pulling is used as a means of regulating emotions in persons with trichotillomania.

The ComB Model also provides for positive feedback derived from achievement of personal goals. These personal goals may be cognitively driven and mediated by affect. In this view, thoughts such as "these gray hairs must go" lead to strong negative feelings (e.g., irritation, disgust) upon detection of the unwanted hairs; removal of these hairs results in feelings of satisfaction.

Another phenomenon associated with trichotillomania, in which affect may play a significant role, occurs in patients who report a dissociative-like state associated with hair-pulling binges. Some trichotillomania patients describe a "tunnel vision" or "zoning out" experience during some episodes, in which they are lost in their pulling. Whether this serves an escape function from unwanted feelings warrants further investigation, as does the possibility that this phenomenon represents a link between trichotillomania and childhood trauma in some patients (Lochner et al. 2004).

AVERSIVE CONSEQUENCES OF HAIR PULLING

Although the ComB Model emphasizes consequences that foster and maintain hair pulling, it also identifies varieties of aversive consequences that may discourage further pulling within a given episode. Among these are undesired emotional states, such as anxiety, shame, and depressed mood, and other aversive experiences such as pain, discomfort, bleeding, or fatigue. Trichotillomania subjects interviewed in Diefenbach et al.'s (2002) study reported guilt, sadness, and anxiety after pulling episodes.

Beyond the broad range of phenomena associated with trichotillomania identified and organized within the ComB Model, the disorder often involves an array of personal, emotional, and interpersonal problems that lie outside the parameters of the model. Besides the cosmetic damage of hair loss, ranging from imperceptible thinning to obvious patchiness, with total baldness or denuding at the extreme, a variety of medical conditions can also be associated with trichotillomania. Damage to the skin may occur at pulling sites, especially if sharp implements are employed, with infections and scarring sometimes occurring. Changes in hair color and texture, either temporary or permanent, have been noted with recurrent pulling. Hair color can change to white or gray, and hair can become increasingly thick and curly (Christenson and Mansueto 1999).

In addition, psychological suffering as a consequence of trichotillomania is typical and can be intense. The degree of suffering may be underestimated by others, including clinicians, thereby adding further distress to hair pullers. The self-inflicted and apparently "voluntary" nature of their pulling can lead to the incorrect assumption that they have the ability to end the hair pulling if they "really want to" (O'Sullivan et al. 2000). The high proportion of emotional suffering experienced by trichotillomania patients was reported by Mansueto (1991) and has been largely corroborated in subsequent research (Stemberger et al. 2000).

Interpersonally generated emotional distress associated with trichotillomania often leads to efforts to conceal cosmetic damage with camouflaging hairstyles, makeup, clothing, hairpieces, and other devices (Mansueto 1991). Efforts to maintain secrecy about the problem cause patients to avoid a host of everyday activities that others take for granted. Table 1–4 illustrates the activities avoided by hair pullers in Stemberger et al.'s (2000) sample.

Physical problems can also occur in some individuals with trichotillomania. Repetitive motions and strained postures in some hair pullers can result in musculoskeletal injury, manifesting as back, shoulder, neck, and hand pain. Dental damage can result from oral activity with hairs and can produce worn or broken teeth, and intestinal problems can occur if substantial amounts of hair are swallowed. Furthermore, avoidance of routine and necessary health care may occur because many hair pullers fear that their trichotillomania might be detected under close scrutiny (O'Sullivan et al. 2000).

The broad view of trichotillomania and of its associated problems suggests that the impact of this disorder can be severe, pervasive, and incapacitating. The large Internet-based survey of individuals with self-reported symptoms documented the social, occupational, and academic impact of the disorder (Woods et al. 2006). In that sample, subjects reported that hair pulling moderately interfered with home management tasks, their social lives, and their ability to maintain close relationships with others. Moreover, hair pulling had a mild impact on their ability to work and a mild to moderate impact on academic functioning. In a similar Internet-based survey of 130 youths ages 10–17 years with self- and parent-reported trichotillomania symptoms, mild to moderate functional impairment in social and academic functioning was reported, as well as elevated anxiety and depressive symptoms (Franklin et al. 2008).

Not all hair pullers experience significant impairment in functioning, however. Mansueto et al. (2007) studied hair pulling in 248 African American college students. Among the 63% who reported pulling hair, none reported negative functional impact as a consequence of hair pulling. A lower degree of hair-pulling severity in that sample may account for these findings, however; anecdotal evidence suggests that trichotillomania can have life-altering effects and may severely impair the functionality and life satisfaction of some hair pullers. Evidence of a significant relationship between psychosocial functioning and hair-pulling severity seems reasonable and has been reported by Diefenbach et al. (2005).

TABLE 1–4. Activities avoided by hair pullers

Activity	Percentage of sample reporting avoidance
Haircuts	63
Swimming	62
Being outside in the wind	42
Sports	35
Sexual intimacy	35
Lighted areas	25
Public activities	22

Source. Data derived from the findings of Stemberger et al. (2000).

CONCLUSION

Two decades of advances in our understanding of hair pulling have substantially clarified the picture. Trichotillomania is a relatively common disorder of notable heterogeneity and phenomenological complexity that is frequently accompanied by significant behavioral, emotional, and interpersonal sequelae. The understanding that trichotillomania is not uncommon and that it induces suffering means that increasing efforts to comprehend its nature, treat it effectively, and even prevent its occurrence are warranted.

The degree of heterogeneity and clinical complexity described in this chapter suggests that a search for meaningful, homogeneous subtypes is justified (Lochner et al. 2010), both to further comprehend the nature of the disorder and to aid the development of more effective treatments. In the current state of the science, given the heterogeneity and clinical complexity described here, it seems reasonable to pursue the development of treatments flexible enough to address the diverse and idiosyncratic features that constitute each individual's trichotillomania (e.g., Mansueto et al. 1999).

REFERENCES

American Psychiatric Association: Diagnostic and Statistical Manual of Mental Disorders, 4th Edition, Text Revision. Washington, DC, American Psychiatric Association, 2000

Azrin NH, Nunn RG: Habit reversal: a method of eliminating nervous habits and tics. Behav Res Ther 11:619–628, 1973

Christenson GA: Trichotillomania: from prevalence to comorbidity. Psychiatr Times 12:44–48, 1995

Christenson GA, Mackenzie TB: Trichotillomania, in Handbook of Prescriptive Treatment for Adults. Edited by Herson M, Ammerman RT. New York, Plenum, 1994, pp 217–235

Christenson GA, Mansueto CS: Trichotillomania: descriptive characteristics and phenomenology, in Trichotillomania. Edited by Stein DJ, Christenson GA, Hollander E. Washington, DC, American Psychiatric Press, 1999, pp 1–41

Christenson GA, Mackenzie TB, Mitchell JE: Characteristics of 60 adult chronic hair pullers. Am J Psychiatry 148:365–370, 1991a

Christenson GA, Pyle RL, Mitchell JE: Estimated lifetime prevalence of trichotillomania in college students. J Clin Psychiatry 52:415–417, 1991b

Christenson GA, Ristvedt SL, Mackenzie TB: Identification of trichotillomania cue profiles. Behav Res Ther 31:315–320, 1993

Christenson GA, Mackenzie TB, Mitchell JE: Adult men and women with trichotillomania: a comparison of male and female characteristics. Psychosomatics 35:142–149, 1994

Diefenbach GJ, Mouton-Odum S, Stanley MA: Affective correlates of trichotillomania. Behav Res Ther 40:1305–1316, 2002

Diefenbach GJ, Tolin DF, Hannan S, et al: Trichotillomania: impact on psychosocial functioning and quality of life. Behav Res Ther 43:869–884, 2005

Duke DC, Bodzin DK, Tavares P, et al: The phenomenology of hair pulling in a community sample. J Anxiety Disord 23:1118–1125, 2009

Duke DC, Keeley ML, Geffken GR, et al: Trichotillomania: a current review. Clin Psychol Rev 30:181–193, 2010

Flessner CA, Conelea CA, Woods DW, et al: Styles of pulling in trichotillomania: exploring differences in symptom severity, phenomenology, and functional impact. Behav Res Ther 46:345–357, 2008

Flessner CA, Woods DW, Franklin ME, et al: Cross-sectional study of women with trichotillomania: a preliminary examination of pulling styles, severity, phenomenology, and functional impact. Child Psychiatry Hum Dev 40:153–167, 2009

Franklin ME, Flessner CA, Woods DW, et al: The child and adolescent trichotillomania impact project: descriptive psychopathology, comorbidity, functional impairment, and treatment utilization. J Dev Behav Pediatr 29:493–500, 2008

Grant JE, Christenson GA: Examination of gender in pathologic grooming behaviors. Psychiatr Q 78:259–267, 2007

Grant JE, Odlaug BL: Clinical characteristics of trichotillomania with trichophagia. Compr Psychiatry 49:579–584, 2008

Grant JE, Levine L, Kim D, et al: Impulse control disorders in adult psychiatric inpatients. Am J Psychiatry 162:2184–2188, 2005

Keuthen NJ, O'Sullivan RL, Hayday CF, et al: The relationship of menstrual cycle and pregnancy to compulsive hairpulling. Psychother Psychosom 66:33–37, 1997

Keuthen NJ, O'Sullivan RL, Jefferys DE: Trichotillomania: clinical concepts and treatment approaches, in Obsessive-Compulsive Disorders: Practical Management, 3rd Edition. Edited by Jenike MA, Baer L, Minichiello WE. Chicago, IL, Mosby, 1998, pp 162–186

Keuthen NJ, Fraim C, Deckersbach TD, et al: Longitudinal follow-up of naturalistic treatment outcome in patients with trichotillomania. J Clin Psychiatry 62:101–107, 2001

King RA, Xohar AH, Ratzoni G, et al: An epidemiological study of trichotillomania in Israeli adolescents. J Am Acad Child Adolesc Psychiatry 34:1212–1215, 1995

Lochner C, Seedat S, Hemmings SM, et al: Dissociative experiences in obsessive-compulsive disorder and trichotillomania: clinical and genetic findings. Compr Psychiatry 45:384–391, 2004

Lochner C, Seedat S, Stein DJ: Chronic hair-pulling: phenomenology-based subtypes. J Anxiety Disord 24:196–202, 2010

Mackenzie TB, Ristvedt SL, Christenson GA, et al: Identification of cues associated with compulsive, bulimic, and hair-pulling symptoms. J Behav Ther Exp Psychiatry 26:9–16, 1995

Mansueto CS: Trichotillomania in focus. OCD Newsletter 5:10–11, 1991

Mansueto CS, Stemberger RMT, Thomas AM, et al: Trichotillomania: a comprehensive behavioral model. Clin Psychol Rev 17:567–577, 1997

Mansueto CS, Golomb RG, Thomas AM, et al: A comprehensive model for behavioral treatment of trichotillomania. Cogn Behav Pract 6:23–43, 1999

Mansueto CS, Thomas AM, Brice AL: Hair pulling and its affective correlates in an African American university sample. J Anxiety Disord 21:590–599, 2007

McCarley NG, Spirrison CL, Ceminsky JL: Hair pulling behavior reported by African American and non–African American college students. J Psychopathol Behav Assess 24:139–144, 2002

Mehregan AH: Trichotillomania: a clinicopathologic study. Arch Dermatol 102:129–133, 1970

Meunier SA, Tolin DF, Franklin M: Affective and sensory correlates of hair pulling in pediatric trichotillomania. Behav Modif 33:396–407, 2009

Murphy C, Redenius R, O'Neill E, et al: Sleep-isolated trichotillomania: a survey of dermatologists. J Clin Sleep Med 3:719–721, 2007

Neal-Barnett A, Stadulis R: Affective states and racial identity among African American women with trichotillomania. J Natl Med Assoc 98:753–757, 2006

O'Sullivan RL, Keuthen NJ, Christenson GA, et al: Trichotillomania: behavioral symptom or clinical syndrome? Am J Psychiatry 154:1442–1449, 1997

O'Sullivan RL, Mansueto CS, Lerner EA, et al: Characterization of trichotillomania: a phenomenological model with clinical relevance to obsessive-compulsive spectrum disorders. Psychiatr Clin North Am 23:587–604, 2000

Penzel F: The Hair-Pulling Problem: A Complete Guide to Trichotillomania. New York, Oxford University Press, 2003

Reeve E: Hair pulling in children and adolescents, in Trichotillomania. Edited by Stein DJ, Christenson GA, Hollander E. Washington, DC, American Psychiatric Press, 1999, pp 201–224

Rothbaum BO, Shaw L, Morris R, et al: Prevalence of trichotillomania in a college freshman population. J Clin Psychiatry 54:72–73, 1993

Schachter M: Zum Problem der kindlichen trichotillomanie. Praxis der Kinderpsychologie und Kinderpsychiatrie 10:120–124, 1961

Shusterman A, Feld L, Baer L, et al: Affective regulation in trichotillomania: evidence from a large-scale internet survey. Behav Res Ther 47:637–644, 2009

Stanley MA, Borden JW, Bell GE, et al: Nonclinical hair pulling: phenomenology and related psychopathology. J Anxiety Disord 8:119–130, 1994

Stemberger RMT, Thomas AM, Mansueto CS, et al: Personal toll of trichotillomania: behavioral and interpersonal sequelae. J Anxiety Disord 14:97–104, 2000

Swedo SE, Rapoport JL: Annotation: trichotillomania. J Child Psychol Psychiatry 32:401–409, 1991

Szepietowski JC, Salomon J, Pacan P, et al: Frequency and treatment of trichotillomania in Poland. Acta Derm Venereol 89:267–270, 2009

Walsh KH, McDougle CJ: Trichotillomania: presentation, etiology, diagnosis and therapy. Am J Clin Dermatol 2:327–333, 2001

Woods DW, Flessner CA, Franklin ME, et al: The Trichotillomania Impact Project (TIP): exploring phenomenology, functional impairment, and treatment utilization. J Clin Psychiatry 67:1877–1888, 2006

Wright HH, Holmes GR: Trichotillomania (hair pulling) in toddlers. Psychol Rep 92:228–230, 2003

Chapter 2

PATHOLOGICAL SKIN PICKING

Brian L. Odlaug, B.A.
Jon E. Grant, M.D., M.P.H., J.D.

Pathological skin picking (PSP) is a disorder currently included as an impulse-control disorder not otherwise specified in DSM-IV-TR (American Psychiatric Association 2000). As of yet, agreed-upon diagnostic criteria for PSP are lacking, although criteria based on the phenomenological and psychobiological similarities of PSP to other impulse-control disorders have been proposed (Tables 2–1 and 2–2). The elements common to all the proposed criteria are recurrent and repetitive picking of the skin resulting in noticeable tissue damage, and significant impairment or distress resulting from the picking.

HISTORY

Erasmus Wilson, in 1875, first coined the term *neurotic excoriation* (Wilson 1875) to describe excessive picking behaviors in neurotic patients that were extremely difficult, if not impossible, to control (Adamson 1913, 1915; Pusey and Senear 1920). In 1898, the French dermatologist M.L. Brocq was the first to describe in detail the excoriation of acne in young, "pale, rather feeble girls" who worsened their skin lesions through repetitive picking and scratching (Brocq 1898). Pickers in the early literature were viewed in a nonsympathetic manner, often referred to as "anger-repressing" (Michelson 1945), "highly sensitive" (Seitz 1951), "hostile" and "vindictive" (Zaidens 1951) individuals with a "nervous temperament" (Adamson 1913) and an innate in-

---

TABLE 2–1.   **Proposed diagnostic criteria for pathological skin picking**

Stein et al. 2010

1. Recurrent skin picking resulting in skin lesions.
2. Picking causes clinically significant distress or impairment in social, occupational, or other important areas of functioning.
3. The disturbance is not limited to skin picking due to the primary symptoms of another mental disorder (e.g., fixed beliefs about skin infestation in delusional disorder, perceived defects or flaws in physical appearance in an individual with body dysmorphic disorder), and not due to the direct physiological effects of a substance (e.g., during amphetamine intoxication) or a general medical condition (e.g., dermatological problem).

Keuthen et al. 2010

1. Picking causing tissue damage.
2. Picking not accounted for by other medical or psychiatric illness.
3. Picking causes clinically significant distress or impairment in social, occupational, or other important areas of functioning.

Arnold et al. 2001

1. Recurrent and repetitive picking of the skin resulting in noticeable tissue damage.
2. Preoccupation with or experience of urges to pick skin that is reported as intrusive.
3. Reported feelings of tension, anxiety, or agitation immediately preceding the picking episode.
4. Feelings of pleasure, relief, or satisfaction during picking.
5. The picking cannot be accounted for by another medical (e.g., scabies, eczema) or mental (e.g., cocaine or amphetamine use disorders, parasitosis) disorder.
6. Significant social or occupational impairment results from the picking behavior.

---

ability to relate to others (Zaidens 1951). Picking was described as a response to an "overzealous mother" who drove her daughter to focus on her appearance and subsequently pick at imperfections of the skin (Wrong 1954). These "cunning" individuals with excoriative and uncontrolled picking behavior were not to be trusted, and only through extensive experience on the part of the clinician could the disease be recognized (through facial tremors and nervous mannerisms) and treated appropriately (Stokes and Garner 1929).

Although limited, early medical writings attempted to understand how this pathological form of skin picking differed from other behaviors described by

TABLE 2–2. Comparison of proposed diagnostic criteria for pathological skin picking

	Arnold et al. 2001	Keuthen et al. 2010	Stein et al. 2010
Recurrent picking causing tissue damage	x	x	x
Intrusive preoccupation or urges to pick skin	x		
Tension, anxiety, or agitation immediately preceding picking	x		
Distress or psychosocial impairment resulting from picking	x	x	x
Pleasure or satisfaction resulting from picking	x		
Picking not accounted for by other medical or psychiatric illness[a]	x	x	x

[a]Body dysmorphic disorder, amphetamine use, and dermatological conditions.

dermatologists and psychiatrists. The self-acknowledged nature of the picking behavior and lack of delusionality helped to differentiate PSP from other psychiatric (i.e., delusions of parasitosis or personality disorders) or dermatological (i.e., dermatitis artefacta or dermatitis factitia) conditions that often involve mutilation of the skin (MacKee 1920; Stokes and Garner 1929).

EPIDEMIOLOGY

Although large studies documenting the prevalence of PSP within the general population have yet to be conducted, recent research suggests that the prevalence rate of PSP may be as high as 5.4% in the general population (*n*=354) (Hayes et al. 2009). A recent telephone survey of 2,511 adults found that 16.6% picked their skin to the extent that noticeable tissue damage resulted (Keuthen et al. 2010). When more stringent criteria, including associated distress or functional impairment caused by the picking, were considered in this same sample, however, only 1.4% met the criteria for lifetime PSP (Keuthen et al. 2010). Smaller studies in college students (sample sizes ranging from 105 to 439) have found lifetime prevalence rates of 2.7%–4% (Bohne et al. 2002; Keuthen et al. 2000; Teng et al. 2002).

Clinical samples demonstrate a wide range of prevalence rates (Table 2–3). In a large study of dermatology patients (N=4,576), Griesemer (1978) found that 2% had lifetime PSP. In a study of 102 adolescent psychiatric inpatients with a range of primary disorders, 11.8% also met the criteria for current PSP (Grant et al. 2007b). High lifetime rates of PSP have been found in individuals with body dysmorphic disorder (BDD; 26.8%–44.9%) as well as in adolescents (12.8%) and adults (10.8%) with obsessive-compulsive disorder (OCD) (Grant et al. 2006a, 2006b, 2010a; Phillips and Taub 1995).

As noted, discrepancies between reported prevalence rates of PSP have been large, and although epidemiological data are growing, significant limitations remain. These limitations include the relatively small sample sizes and the lack of agreed-upon operational definitions and diagnostic criteria. Table 2–3 illustrates the prevalence studies that have been conducted, including the method of assessment and subject cohort (i.e., clinical or general population).

CLINICAL CHARACTERISTICS

Age at Onset

PSP appears to have a trimodal age at onset, occurring before age 10 years, in adolescence or young adulthood (ages 15–21), and then again between the ages of 30 and 45, although onset in childhood or adolescence appears to be most common (Arnold et al. 1998, 1999; Bohne et al. 2002; Calikusu et al. 2003; Keuthen et al. 2000, 2007; Odlaug and Grant 2007; Simeon et al. 1997). A sample of 372 PSP subjects recruited through an Internet-based treatment program had a mean age at onset of 14.4 years (Flessner et al. 2007a), whereas another sample of 29 treatment-seeking individuals had a mean age at onset of 13.2±8.1 years (Keuthen et al. 2007). Similarly, a treatment-seeking sample of 21 individuals had an average age at onset of 16.1± 9.0 years (Simeon et al. 1997), whereas another treatment study found age at onset to be 15.3±13.8 years (Grant et al. 2007a).

This apparent trimodal onset of PSP has led researchers to investigate whether there may be discrete phenomenological differences between early- and later-onset PSP. A study of 40 individuals with PSP sought to examine this question and separated individuals based on age at onset. Of 40 individuals with PSP, 19 (47.5%) reported an age at onset before 10 years of age (mean age at onset, 5.6±2.2 years) and 21 (52.5%) reported onset after 10 years of age (mean age at onset, 20.3±11.6 years). Clinically, the two groups were very similar, although the later-onset group reported spending more time picking each day (mean, 79.8±23.3 vs. 60.6±33.1 minutes), whereas

TABLE 2–3. Prevalence of pathological skin picking (PSP) in community and clinical samples

Study	Prevalence of PSP, %	Sample size, N	Mean age, y; % female	Method of assessment	Criteria used to define PSP	Place of assessment (i.e., sample)
Keuthen et al. 2010	1.4	2,511	41.9; 76.5%	Random-digit dialing	1) Noticeable tissue damage 2) Distress 3) Not accounted for by medical condition	Community sample
Griesemer 1978	2.0	4,576	Not specified	Direct interview	Not specified	Dermatology clinic patients and hospital-based community sample
Bohne et al. 2002	2.3	133	Mean age of PSP subjects not specified; overall=22; 100%	Survey distributed in undergraduate psychology class	1) Noticeable tissue damage 2) Significant functional impairment 3) Not accounted for by medical condition	Collegiate student sample

TABLE 2–3.   Prevalence of pathological skin picking (PSP) in community and clinical samples (*continued*)

Study	Prevalence of PSP, %	Sample size, N	Mean age, y; % female	Method of assessment	Criteria used to define PSP	Place of assessment (i.e., sample)
Teng et al. 2002	2.7	439	Mean age of PSP subjects not specified/ overall=20.9; 83.3%	Survey distributed in undergraduate psychology class	1) Engaged in picking >5× a day for at least 4 weeks 2) Picking caused injury or interfered with functioning	Collegiate student sample
Keuthen et al. 2000	3.8	105	21.3; 100%	Survey distributed in undergraduate psychology class	1) Noticeable tissue damage 2) Significant functional impairment	Collegiate student sample
Hayes et al. 2009	5.4	354	Mean age and gender of PSP subjects not specified/ overall=32.3; 56.8%	Direct interview	1) Noticeable tissue damage 2) Significant functional impairment	Community sample
Grant et al. 2006a	8.9	293	Mean age and gender of PSP subjects not specified/overall=40.6; 56.8%	Direct interview	Based on DSM-IV-TR criteria for impulse-control disorders such as trichotillomania	OCD patients

TABLE 2–3. Prevalence of pathological skin picking (PSP) in community and clinical samples (*continued*)

Study	Prevalence of PSP, %	Sample size, N	Mean age, y; % female	Method of assessment	Criteria used to define PSP	Place of assessment (i.e., sample)
Grant et al. 2007b	11.8	102	Mean age of PSP subjects not specified/ overall = 15.8; 75%	Direct interview	Arnold et al. 2001	Adolescent psychiatric inpatients
Cullen et al. 2001	24.0	75	34.1; 61.1%	Direct interview	Arnold et al. 2001	OCD patients
Phillips and Taub 1995	26.8	123	30.5; 57.6%	Direct interview	Picking at the skin "excessively"	BDD patients
Grant et al. 2006b	44.9	176	30.5; 82.3%	Direct interview	1) Picking >1 hour each day 2) Significant functional impairment	BDD patients

Note. BDD=body dysmorphic disorder; OCD=obsessive–compulsive disorder.

the childhood-onset group was less likely to have ever received treatment for picking (Odlaug and Grant 2007).

Adolescents and young adults often report onset of picking associated with a dermatological illness such as acne (Wilhelm et al. 1999; Wrong 1954). A study of 92 subjects with PSP found that 5 (5.4%) reported picking after the onset of a medical condition (although the condition was not specified) (Flessner and Woods 2006). Other studies, however, have reported that picking onset did not coincide with a medical condition but instead *resulted* in medical problems. Simeon et al. (1997) found that 15 (71.4%) of the 21 subjects enrolled in a treatment study picked at "normal" skin. This percentage is similar to the 51.6% of subjects in another treatment study who reported picking at normal skin (Wilhelm et al. 1999). The differences between groups who pick at medically compromised skin versus those who pick at normal, unaffected skin, however, are unknown at this time and merit exploration.

Course of Illness

Although the course of illness may vary, PSP is most often considered to be a chronic disorder that tends to fluctuate in intensity over time (Gupta et al. 1986, 1987; Phillips and Taub 1995). Samples of treatment-seeking individuals have illustrated the chronic course of PSP, and one study found that subjects had a mean duration of illness of 25.1 ± 9.1 years (Bloch et al. 2001). Other studies (with sample sizes of 21–31 subjects) have reported similar durations of illness (18–21 years) (Grant et al. 2007a; Keuthen et al. 2007; Simeon et al. 1997; Wilhelm et al. 1999).

Shorter, yet still significant, durations of illness have also been noted for PSP. Arnold et al. (1998) found a mean duration of 8 ± 10 years for their sample of 32 PSP patients, whereas a later study of 14 subjects (Arnold et al. 2001) found a mean duration of 6.2 ± 6.6 years. Most studies, regardless of duration of illness, report that the severity of picking waxes and wanes over time (Simeon et al. 1997).

Clinical Presentation

Although the specific diagnostic criteria for PSP have yet to be agreed upon, the hallmark characteristic is clearly the recurrent picking at one's own skin, resulting in tissue damage. Whereas most early descriptions of PSP in the literature emphasized the mechanistic simplicity of picking, more recent reports have highlighted both the phenomenological complexity and the possible heterogeneity of the disorder (Grant and Odlaug 2009).

A significant amount of time is expended each day picking, with many subjects reporting that the picking behavior is "compulsive" (Fruensgaard 1984) and occupies several hours each day (Arnold et al. 1998; Bloch et al. 2001;

Flessner and Woods 2006; Grant et al. 2007a). One study of 92 individuals reported that patients spent, on average, 2.8 hours per day resisting the urge to pick, thinking about picking, or picking (Flessner and Woods 2006). Another study of 34 PSP patients found that 5 (15%) picked for more than 3 hours each day and 5 (15%) picked for more than 8 hours daily (Arnold et al. 1998). Because of the amount of time spent picking, patients often miss work or school (Arnold et al. 2001; Flessner and Woods 2006), and 51.1% of students and 34.4% of workers report that picking affects their daily scholastic or occupational functioning (Flessner and Woods 2006).

Although the face is the most commonly reported site of picking, other areas frequently picked include the fingers, torso, arms, legs, back, pubic area, and feet (Arnold et al. 1998; Bloch et al. 2001; Flessner and Woods 2006; Grant et al. 2007a; Odlaug and Grant 2008a, 2008b; Wilhelm et al. 1999) (Table 2–4). Additionally, many individuals report having a primary area of picking but frequently pick at other sites on the body in order to allow the most significantly excoriated areas to heal (Arnold et al. 1998; Bohne et al. 2002; Odlaug and Grant 2008a). In fact, 32.6%–100% of patients report picking from multiple sites on the body (Arnold et al. 1998; Bloch et al. 2001; Flessner and Woods 2006; Grant et al. 2007a; Wilhelm et al. 1999). A study of 60 individuals with PSP found that subjects picked from a mean of 2.3 ± 1.2 sites on the body (Odlaug and Grant 2008a). Although fingernails are most commonly used to pick, patients also report using knives, scissors, tweezers, pins, letter openers, and other objects to excoriate the skin (Arnold et al. 1998; Bloch et al. 2001; Grant et al. 2007a; Odlaug and Grant 2008b).

Gratifying experiences have the potential to serve as reinforcing events. Many individuals with PSP experience forms of relief or gratification associated with picking (Bloch et al. 2001), although such relief does not occur in all individuals. Additionally, distinctly pleasurable feelings are often a result of the picking and have been reported in 52%–79% of individuals with PSP (Arnold et al. 1998; Keuthen et al. 2010; Simeon et al. 1997), thus providing potentially positively reinforcing consequences for the behavior. Another type of gratification occurs when picking functions to eliminate aversive sensations that exist prior to picking (i.e., the sensation that the skin has a bump or that something is "not right" about the feel of the skin).

Skin picking may function to regulate affective states and nervous system arousal (Neziroglu et al. 2008). Many individuals report picking in the morning before leaving the home or at bedtime to soothe or calm themselves (Wilhelm et al. 1999). Skin picking may therefore regulate a range of affective states, such as anxiety, depression, and fatigue (Simeon et al. 1997). Individuals with PSP endorsing these negative affective states also report focused picking behavior, similar to the emotions that trigger hair pulling in trichotillomania (Flessner et al. 2007b; Walther et al. 2009).

The psychological consequences of PSP are typical and can be intense. The degree of suffering may be underestimated by others, including clinicians, thereby adding further distress. A recent study assessing self-reported quality of life in 59 PSP and 70 trichotillomania subjects compared with 25 healthy control subjects found that PSP subjects reported significantly higher rates of psychosocial dysfunction and a lower overall quality of life compared with trichotillomania and control subjects (Odlaug et al. 2010a). PSP subjects were also significantly less likely to have received formal treatment and spent more time engaging in the behavior each day (mean, 120 minutes) compared with trichotillomania subjects (mean, 45 minutes).

Emotional distress associated with PSP often leads to efforts to conceal cosmetic damage. Studies have found that 68%–85% of subjects report using some form of concealment to hide significantly excoriated areas of the skin (Arnold et al. 1998; Bohne et al. 2002; Flessner and Woods 2006). The most commonly reported concealment methods include using makeup (44.6%) and clothing (e.g., wearing long-sleeved shirts and pants instead of short-sleeved shirts and shorts, even with great discomfort in hot weather [40.2%]) (Flessner and Woods 2006). One study found that PSP patients spent, on average, $160 per year on products to conceal the effects of their picking (Flessner and Woods 2006). This camouflaging of the body is similar to behaviors seen in other psychiatric disorders, such as BDD. The similarities and differences between PSP and disorders such as BDD, however, are discussed later in this chapter.

Efforts to maintain secrecy about the problem cause individuals with PSP to avoid a host of everyday activities that others take for granted. Patients often report avoiding social activities, confining themselves to their homes, and even skipping vacations as a result of their embarrassment (Arnold et al. 1998; Flessner and Woods 2006).

Triggers to Picking

Many, but not all, individuals who pick their skin report an impulse or urge to pick that precedes picking episodes (Bloch et al. 2001). In such cases, the urges tend to occur within specific circumstances and in response to specific cues. These circumstances and cues can vary greatly both between and within individuals with PSP. Looking at (26.7%–87%) or feeling (44%–94%) the skin is generally reported as the most common trigger to picking (Arnold et al. 1998; Odlaug and Grant 2008a; Wilhelm et al. 1999), although "downtime," boredom, feeling tired, and stress have all been endorsed as triggering a picking episode (Doran et al. 1985; Hajcak et al. 2006; Neziroglu et al. 2008; Odlaug and Grant 2008a). Most patients report picking only when they are alone (Arnold et al. 1998; Grant et al. 2007a; Wilhelm et al. 1999). In

TABLE 2–4. Body sites involved in pathological skin picking, by sample percentage

	Simeon et al. 1997 (N=21)	Arnold et al. 1998 (N=34)	Wilhelm et al. 1999 (N=31[a])	Bloch et al. 2001 (N=15)	Flessner and Woods 2006 (N=92)	Grant et al. 2007a (N=24[b])	Grant et al. 2010b (N=32[b])
Multiple sites	23.8	82.0	100	46.7	32.6	83.3	75.0
Face	33.3	50	98	60	65.2	45.8[b]	46.9[b]
Head (scalp)	9.5	24	58	13.3	17.4		
Hands[c]	14.3	26.5	55	40	27.2	54.2[b]	40.6[b]
Arms	9.5	47	48	20	51.1	45.8[b]	9.4[b]
Legs	4.8	29	42	26.7	40.2		
Feet	—	—	—	—	19.6		
Torso	—	12	55	—	21.7	20.8	3.1
Back	4.8	18	67	6.7	27.2	—	—
Pubic area	—	12	—	—	6.5	—	—
Buttocks	—	9	—	—	—	—	—

[a]Numbers are approximations based on table provided in Wilhelm et al. 1999 text.
[b]Study combined face/head, feet/hands, and arms/legs.
[c]Includes cuticles.

such cases, individuals often report increasing tension throughout the day and looking forward to picking as soon as they arrive home for the evening.

In addition to triggers to pick, which vary widely within and between individuals with PSP, the overall awareness of picking behavior by those with PSP also varies. Individuals who are generally unaware of their picking (i.e., 50% aware) are considered "automatic" or "habitual" pickers compared with people generally conscious of engaging in the behavior, who are referred to as "focused" pickers. A treatment study of 24 subjects found that 16 (66.7%) were aware of their picking behavior at least 50% of the time, whereas the other 8 (33.3%) picked unconsciously or "automatically" the majority of the time (Grant et al. 2007a). This is similar to the 73.9% of subjects reporting being aware of their picking at least 50% of the time in a sample of 40 individuals with PSP (Neziroglu et al. 2008). These percentages, however, differ from the 76% of patients in a study of 34 subjects with PSP who reported that they often "found" themselves picking—a more habitual form of picking (Arnold et al. 1998).

This variance of awareness within PSP patients is similar to the focused versus automatic pulling behavior noted in trichotillomania (Christenson and Mackenzie 1994; see also Chapter 1, "Trichotillomania: Epidemiology and Clinical Characteristics"). A comparison of 21 patients with PSP compared with 68 patients with trichotillomania found that trichotillomania patients had significantly higher rates of "dissociative" behavior, meaning that pickers might be more focused and engaged in their behavior compared with trichotillomania patients (Lochner et al. 2002). The clinical similarities and differences between subtypes of automatic versus focused picking have not been examined extensively, although scales to capture these two subtypes of skin picking have been developed (Walther et al. 2009).

GENDER DIFFERENCES

In most surveys of adults, PSP appears to occur much more frequently in females (83.3%–94.1%) (Arnold et al. 2001; Ehsani et al. 2009; Flessner et al. 2007a; Grant et al. 2007a, 2010b; Teng et al. 2002; Wilhelm et al. 1999). The predominance of females seen in samples of PSP subjects is similar to the 90%–92.3% female preponderance seen in other grooming disorders, such as trichotillomania (Grant et al. 2009; Woods et al. 2006). Although arguably more common in females, skin picking is not exclusively a female problem. Bohne et al. (2002) surveyed 133 undergraduate students and found that men and women had similar rates of picking (although the specific gender difference was not detailed). Although picking is not uncommon in males, picking that causes tissue damage appears to occur much more frequently in females.

A recent community study examining picking behaviors in 354 adults found that females were much more likely to engage in clinically significant picking behavior (15.0%) compared with males (6.1%) (Hayes et al. 2009). Females were also significantly more likely to have anxiety, depressive symptoms, and more severe skin picking (Hayes et al. 2009). A study of 77 individuals (65 [84.4%] of whom were female) with either PSP or trichotillomania found that males and females overall were clinically similar but that men were more likely to have a co-occurring anxiety disorder, a later age at onset, and more severe functional impairment (Grant and Christenson 2007).

Various theories have been proposed to explain why females appear more likely to have PSP. One theory is that PSP may be equally common in men and women but that women are simply more likely to seek professional help (Bohne et al. 2002). In addition, skin lesions on the face and hands may be less important to men and this may lead men to present for treatment less often than women. An alternative theory is that the gender discrepancy is real and that perhaps hormonal differences play a role in this behavior. One study supporting this theory found PSP symptoms were exacerbated premenstrually (Wilhelm et al. 1999).

MEDICAL COMPLICATIONS

Skin picking often results in significant tissue damage, leading to infections, lesions, or significant scarring (Keuthen et al. 2007; Lyell 1972; Neziroglu et al. 2008; Odlaug and Grant 2008a; Wrong 1954). The affected areas of the body have been described as weeping, scarred, or crusted with post-inflammatory hypo- or hyperpigmentation (Gupta et al. 1987). Further medical complications, such as synovitis of the wrists, have been reported as a result of years of picking (Simeon et al. 1997).

The medical complications of picking can be significant and even life threatening. Arnold et al. (1998) described a subject who had excoriated the skin on the dorsum of the hands so severely that physicians considered amputation. Weintraub et al. (2000) described a 47-year-old patient who developed an epidural abscess and paralysis due to hours of picking each day. Sometimes picking may warrant corrective plastic surgery (Arnold et al. 1998; Neziroglu et al. 2008). Another report documented a patient with severe, life-threatening PSP who required bilateral capsulotomies using gamma knife radiosurgery after several medication trials and skin grafting were unsuccessful (Kondziolka and Hudak 2008). O'Sullivan et al. (1999) described a patient who had picked through the dermis, subcutaneous tissue, and musculature on her neck, eventually exposing the carotid artery—a life-threatening complication.

Despite the medical complications of severe skin picking, seeking medical help from a physician is uncommon (Grant et al. 2007a). In fact, some studies have indicated that less than 20% of subjects seek treatment for their picking (Flessner and Woods 2006; Grant et al. 2007a). In a study of 31 patients with PSP, only 14 (45%) had ever sought any treatment (Wilhelm et al. 1999). Individuals with PSP often report being unaware that treatments are available or, more alarmingly, that PSP is a disorder at all (Grant et al. 2007a).

COMORBIDITY

Psychiatric comorbidity is the rule, not the exception, for individuals with PSP. Lifetime rates of DSM-IV Axis I disorders have been found to occur in 54.5%–100% of individuals with PSP (Arnold et al. 1998; Mutasim and Adams 2009; Odlaug and Grant 2007, 2008a, 2008b). High lifetime rates of co-occurring major depressive (12.5%–48%), anxiety (other than OCD; 8%–23%), obsessive-compulsive (6%–68%), bipolar (12%–35.7%), eating (10%–21%), alcohol use (14%–36%), and attention-deficit (9.1%) disorders have been reported (Arnold et al. 1998, 2001; Bloch et al. 2001; Grant et al. 2007a; Keuthen et al. 2007; Lochner et al. 2002; Mutasim and Adams 2009; Neziroglu et al. 2008; Odlaug and Grant 2007, 2008a, 2008b; Phillips and Taub 1995; Simeon et al. 1997; Wilhelm et al. 1999). Whether the co-occurring disorders share a common pathophysiology with PSP or are simply a result of picking needs further examination. A study of 92 individuals with PSP found that 17.4% used illegal drugs, 22.8% used tobacco products, and 25.0% used alcohol to relieve feelings associated with PSP; additionally, 85.9% of subjects reported anxiety and 66.3% reported depression due to picking (Flessner and Woods 2006).

Other pathological grooming disorders (trichotillomania and compulsive nail biting) are also common in patients with PSP (Arnold et al. 1998; Lochner et al. 2002; Odlaug and Grant 2008b). A study of 60 patients with PSP found lifetime rates of co-occurring trichotillomania of 38.3% and compulsive nail biting of 31.7% (Odlaug and Grant 2008a). These rates are substantially higher than the rates of trichotillomania and compulsive nail biting seen in the general population (0.6%–3.9% and 6.4%–10.1%, respectively) (Christenson et al. 1991; Odlaug et al. 2010b; Woods et al. 1996).

Reports have also indicated substantial comorbidity of PSP with BDD (Arnold et al. 1998; Grant and Odlaug 2009; Grant et al. 2006b; Phillips and Taub 1995). Grant et al. (2006b) found that 44.9% and 36.9% of BDD subjects met lifetime and current criteria for PSP, respectively. An earlier study found that 26.8% of BDD subjects picked their skin secondary to their BDD (Phillips and Taub 1995). Arnold et al. (1998) found that 11 (32%) of their 34 PSP subjects had co-occurring BDD.

The overlap between PSP and BDD highlights the complexity and heterogeneity of PSP. Many patients with BDD pick at their skin to improve their appearance (Phillips 2005), and these individuals may have PSP secondary to BDD. Other individuals with PSP, however, do not pick their skin because of their appearance. In both cases, there is picking but there may in fact be distinct pathophysiologies underlying the picking. Understanding these distinctions may have clinical importance, because the treatments for PSP and BDD often differ (Grant and Odlaug 2009; Phillips 2005).

Axis II personality disorders, although poorly documented in PSP, may be common in PSP. Co-occurring obsessive-compulsive (19.0%–48.4%), borderline (7.5%–33.3%), and avoidant (4.8%–22.6%) personality disorders have been documented (Lochner et al. 2002; Neziroglu et al. 2008; Wilhelm et al. 1999). These personality disorders may complicate treatment and increase the severity of the overall picking.

FAMILY HISTORY

Psychiatric illness appears to be elevated in the first-degree relatives of those with PSP. A sample of 40 subjects with PSP found a lifetime Axis I history in 87.5% ($n=28$) of first-degree relatives, including 43% with skin picking (Neziroglu et al. 2008), whereas another study of 34 PSP patients found lifetime alcoholism in 37.5% of first-degree relatives (Arnold et al. 1998). A study of 31 individuals with PSP found that 45.2% ($n=14$) of first-degree relatives also picked their skin (Wilhelm et al. 1999). These rates are similar to those found in the first-degree relatives of PSP patients in two other studies (19.0%–37.5%) (Grant et al. 2007a; Simeon et al. 1997). Larger samples have found high rates of PSP (28.3%–30.3%) and trichotillomania (6.1%–10.0%) in the first-degree family members of PSP patients (Odlaug and Grant 2008a, 2008b). Although there appears to be a familial link between PSP and several disorders, the question of genetic predisposition to picking behaviors has yet to be resolved.

NEUROBIOLOGY

Animal Models

Animal models represent useful tools to investigate the pathophysiology of PSP. Although these animal models can be used to explain PSP, they could also apply equally well to trichotillomania or even OCD. The existing ethological models focus on spontaneously arising repetitive or stereotypic behaviors, such as tail chasing and fur chewing (Brown et al. 1987; Stein et al.

1994), and behaviors driven by conflict, frustration, or stress, such as grooming, cleaning, and pecking (Stein et al. 1994). Bordnick et al. (1994) presented an avian model of feather picking that may reflect the behaviors of PSP. Birds tend to pluck out their feathers at times of stress or boredom, and feather picking in birds is associated with feather loss or damage to body areas (Moon-Fanelli et al. 1999).

Another candidate model of PSP is the *Hoxb8* knockout mouse. Greer and Capecchi (2002) reported that mice with mutations of the *Hoxb8* gene groomed excessively to the point of skin lesions and hair removal compared with their control counterparts. These mutant mice demonstrated normal cutaneous sensation and no evidence of an inflammatory response was present, suggesting that the behavior was not due to skin abnormalities or abnormalities of the peripheral nervous system. This transgenic model is promising because the excessive grooming of *Hoxb8* mutant mice is similar to the excessive and repetitive grooming behaviors noted in PSP. Furthermore, *Hoxb8* is expressed in the orbital cortex, the anterior cingulate, the striatum, and the limbic system (Hyman 2010).

Cognitive Functioning

Cognitive deficits may be expected in PSP given the often reported comments regarding an inability to stop the picking behavior. The repetitive physical symptoms of PSP suggest underlying dysfunction of motor inhibitory control processes. Motor impulsivity is classically assessed using tasks that require volunteers to make simple motor responses (e.g., pressing a button) on some computer trials but not on others. Stop-signal tasks have been widely validated and shown to be sensitive to impulsivity and right frontal lesions (Aron et al. 2004, 2007; Logan et al. 1984). These tasks measure the ability of subjects to actively inhibit an already triggered motor command. Stop-signal tasks use an individually tailored tracking algorithm to estimate the time taken by the brain to suppress an already initiated response (referred to as the stop-signal reaction time). A recent study of 20 individuals with PSP and 20 healthy control subjects found that subjects with PSP exhibited impaired inhibitory control (i.e., increased stop-signal reaction times) compared with healthy control subjects (Odlaug et al. 2010a). Response inhibition as a cognitive function is dependent on neural circuitry, including the right inferior frontal gyrus (Aron and Poldrack 2005, 2006; Aron et al. 2003). These findings suggest possible inhibitory dysregulation in the pathophysiology of PSP.

CONCLUSION

PSP appears to be a relatively common disorder of notable heterogeneity and phenomenological complexity that is frequently accompanied by significant emotional and physical consequences. Given the heterogeneity of PSP, future research needs to identify subtypes of PSP as a means of better understanding and thereby preventing or treating this disorder. An exploration of the similarities and differences between PSP and other disorders such as trichotillomania, OCD, and BDD must be undertaken to better classify PSP in psychiatric and dermatological settings. From a public health perspective, education about PSP, including its relatively high prevalence in the general population and the medical complications of the behavior, should be disseminated to educational institutions, family practice clinics, and community resource centers. Raising awareness of the behavior may promote the development of effective treatment options to combat this often damaging and chronic condition.

REFERENCES

Adamson HG: Acne urticata (neurotic excoriations—one type). Proc R Soc Med 6:21–22, 1913

Adamson HG: Acne urticata and other forms of neurotic excoriations. Br J Dermatol 27:1–12, 1915

American Psychiatric Association: Diagnostic and Statistical Manual of Mental Disorders, 4th Edition, Text Revision. Washington, DC, American Psychiatric Publishing, 2000

Arnold LM, McElroy SL, Mutasim DF, et al: Characteristics of 34 adults with psychogenic excoriation. J Clin Psychiatry 59:509–514, 1998

Arnold LM, Mutasim DF, Dwight MM, et al: An open clinical trial of fluvoxamine treatment of psychogenic excoriation. J Clin Psychopharmacol 19:15–18, 1999

Arnold LM, Auchenbach MB, McElroy SL: Psychogenic excoriation: clinical features, proposed diagnostic criteria, epidemiology and approaches to treatment. CNS Drugs 15:351–359, 2001

Aron AR, Poldrack RA: The cognitive neuroscience of response inhibition: relevance for genetic research in attention-deficit/hyperactivity disorder. Biol Psychiatry 57:1285–1292, 2005

Aron AR, Poldrack RA: Cortical and subcortical contributions to stop signal response inhibition: role of the subthalamic nucleus. J Neurosci 26:2424–2433, 2006

Aron AR, Fletcher PC, Bullmore ET, et al: Stop-signal inhibition disrupted by damage to right inferior frontal gyrus in humans. Nat Neurosci 6:115–116, 2003

Aron AR, Robbins TW, Poldrack RA: Inhibition and the right inferior frontal cortex. Trends Cogn Sci 8:170–177, 2004

Aron AR, Behrens TE, Smith S, et al: Triangulating a cognitive control network using diffusion-weighted magnetic resonance imaging (MRI) and functional MRI. J Neurosci 27:3743–3752, 2007

Bloch MR, Elliott M, Thompson H, et al: Fluoxetine in pathologic skin-picking: open-label and double-blind results. Psychosomatics 42:314–319, 2001

Bohne A, Wilhelm S, Keuthen NJ, et al: Skin picking in German students: prevalence, phenomenology, and associated characteristics. Behav Modif 26:320–339, 2002

Bordnick PS, Thyer BA, Ritchie BW: Feather picking disorder and trichotillomania: an avian model of human psychopathology. J Behav Ther Exp Psychiatry 25:189–196, 1994

Brocq ML: Acne excoriee of young women and their treatment [in French]. J Pract Rev Gen Clin Ther 12:193–197, 1898

Brown SA, Crowell-Davis S, Malcolm T, et al: Naloxone-responsive compulsive tail chasing in a dog. J Am Vet Med Assoc 190:884–886, 1987

Calikusu C, Yücel B, Polat A, et al: The relation of psychogenic excoriation with psychiatric disorders: a comparative study. Compr Psychiatry 44:256–261, 2003

Christenson GA, Mackenzie TB: Trichotillomania, in Handbook of Prescriptive Treatment for Adults. Edited by Hersen M, Ammerman RT. New York, Plenum, 1994, pp 217–235

Christenson GA, Pyle RL, Mitchell JE: Estimated lifetime prevalence of trichotillomania in college students. J Clin Psychiatry 52:415–417, 1991

Cullen BA, Samuels JF, Bienvenu OJ, et al: The relationship of pathologic skin picking to obsessive-compulsive disorder. J Nerv Ment Dis 189:193–195, 2001

Doran AR, Roy A, Wolkowitz OM: Self-destructive dermatoses. Psychiatr Clin North Am 8:291–298, 1985

Ehsani AH, Toosi S, Mirshams Shahshahani M, et al: Psycho-cutaneous disorders: an epidemiologic study. J Eur Acad Dermatol Venereol 23:945–947, 2009

Flessner CA, Woods DW: Phenomenological characteristics, social problems, and the economic impact associated with chronic skin picking. Behav Modif 30:944–963, 2006

Flessner CA, Mouton-Odum S, Stocker AJ, et al: StopPicking.com: Internet-based treatment for self-injurious skin picking. Dermatol Online J 13:3, 2007a

Flessner CA, Woods DW, Franklin ME, et al: The Milwaukee Inventory for Subtypes of Trichotillomania—Adult Version (MIST-A): development of an instrument for the assessment of "focused" and "automatic" hair pulling. J Psychopathol Behav Assess 30:20–30, 2007b

Fruensgaard K: Neurotic excoriations. A controlled psychiatric evaluation. Acta Psychiatr Scand Suppl 312:1–52, 1984

Grant JE, Christenson GA: Examination of gender in pathologic grooming behaviors. Psychiatr Q 78:259–267, 2007

Grant JE, Odlaug BL: The obsessive-compulsive spectrum and disorders of the skin: a review. Expert Rev Dermatol 4:523–532, 2009

Grant JE, Mancebo MC, Pinto A, et al: Impulse control disorders in adults with obsessive compulsive disorder. J Psychiatr Res 40:494–501, 2006a

Grant JE, Menard W, Phillips KA: Pathological skin picking in individuals with body dysmorphic disorder. Gen Hosp Psychiatry 28:487–493, 2006b

Grant JE, Odlaug BL, Kim SW: Lamotrigine treatment of pathologic skin picking: an open-label study. J Clin Psychiatry 68:1384–1391, 2007a

Grant JE, Williams KA, Potenza MN: Impulse-control disorders in adolescent psychiatric inpatients: co-occurring disorders and sex differences. J Clin Psychiatry 68:1584–1592, 2007b

Grant JE, Odlaug BL, Kim SW: N-Acetylcysteine, a glutamate modulator, in the treatment of trichotillomania: a double-blind, placebo-controlled study. Arch Gen Psychiatry 66:756–763, 2009

Grant JE, Mancebo MC, Eisen JL, et al: Impulse-control disorders in children and adolescents with obsessive-compulsive disorder. Psychiatry Res 175:109–113, 2010a

Grant JE, Odlaug BL, Chamberlain SR, et al: A double-blind, placebo-controlled trial of lamotrigine for pathological skin picking: treatment efficacy and neurocognitive predictors of response. J Clin Psychopharmacol 30:396–403, 2010b

Greer JM, Capecchi MR: Hoxb8 is required for normal grooming behavior in mice. Neuron 33:23–34, 2002

Griesemer RD: Emotionally triggered disease in a dermatologic practice. Psychiatr Ann 8:407–412, 1978

Gupta MA, Gupta AK, Haberman HF: Neurotic excoriations: a review and some new perspectives. Compr Psychiatry 27:381–386, 1986

Gupta MA, Gupta AK, Haberman HF: The self-inflicted dermatoses: a critical review. Gen Hosp Psychiatry 9:45–52, 1987

Hajcak G, Franklin ME, Simons RF, et al: Hairpulling and skin picking in relation to affective distress and obsessive-compulsive symptoms. J Psychopathol Behav Assess 28:177–185, 2006

Hayes SL, Storch EA, Berlanga L: Skin picking behaviors: an examination of the prevalence and severity in a community sample. J Anxiety Disord 23:314–319, 2009

Hyman SE: A bone to pick with compulsive behavior. Cell 141:752–754, 2010

Keuthen NJ, Deckersbach T, Wilhelm S, et al: Repetitive skin picking in a student population and comparison with a sample of self-injurious skin pickers. Psychosomatics 41:210–215, 2000

Keuthen NJ, Jameson M, Loh R, et al: Open-label escitalopram treatment for pathological skin picking. Int Clin Psychopharmacol 22:268–274, 2007

Keuthen NJ, Koran LM, Aboujaoude E, et al: The prevalence of pathologic skin picking in US adults. Compr Psychiatry 51:183–186, 2010

Kondziolka D, Hudak R: Management of obsessive-compulsive disorder–related skin picking with gamma knife radiosurgical anterior capsulotomies: a case report. J Clin Psychiatry 69:1337–1340, 2008

Lochner C, Simeon D, Niehaus DJ, et al: Trichotillomania and skin-picking: a phenomenological comparison. Depress Anxiety 15:83–86, 2002

Logan GD, Cowan WB, Davis KA: On the ability to inhibit simple and choice reaction time responses: a model and a method. J Exp Psychol Hum Percept Perform 10:276–291, 1984

Lyell A: Dermatitis artefacta and self-inflicted disease. Scott Med J 17:187–196, 1972

MacKee GM: Neurotic excoriations. Arch Derm Syphilol 1:256–269, 1920

Michelson HE: Psychosomatic studies in dermatology: the motivation of self-induced eruptions. Arch Derm Syphilol 51:245–250, 1945

Moon-Fanelli AA, Dodman NH, O'Sullivan RI: Veterinary models of compulsive self-grooming: parallels with trichotillomania, in Trichotillomania. Edited by Stein DJ, Christenson GA, Hollander E. Washington, DC, American Psychiatric Press, 1999, pp 63–92

Mutasim DF, Adams BB: The psychiatric profile of patients with psychogenic excoriation. J Am Acad Dermatol 61:611–613, 2009

Neziroglu F, Rabinowitz D, Breytman A, et al: Skin picking phenomenology and severity comparison. Prim Care Companion J Clin Psychiatry 10:306–312, 2008

Odlaug BL, Grant JE: Childhood-onset pathologic skin picking: clinical characteristics and psychiatric comorbidity. Compr Psychiatry 48:388–393, 2007

Odlaug BL, Grant JE: Clinical characteristics and medical complications of pathologic skin picking. Gen Hosp Psychiatry 30:61–66, 2008a

Odlaug BL, Grant JE: Trichotillomania and pathologic skin picking: clinical comparison with an examination of comorbidity. Ann Clin Psychiatry 20:57–63, 2008b

Odlaug BL, Chamberlain SR, Grant JE: Motor inhibition and cognitive flexibility in pathological skin picking. Prog Neuropsychopharmacol Biol Psychiatry 34:208–211, 2010a

Odlaug BL, Grant JE, Kim SW: Quality of life and clinical severity in pathological skin picking and trichotillomania. J Anxiety Disord 24:823–829, 2010b

O'Sullivan RL, Phillips KA, Keuthen NJ, et al: Near-fatal skin picking from delusional body dysmorphic disorder responsive to fluvoxamine. Psychosomatics 40:79–81, 1999

Phillips KA: The Broken Mirror: Understanding and Treating Body Dysmorphic Disorder. New York, Oxford University Press, 2005

Phillips KA, Taub SL: Skin picking as a symptom of body dysmorphic disorder. Psychopharmacol Bull 31:279–288, 1995

Pusey WA, Senear FE: Neurotic excoriations with report of cases. Arch Derm Syphilol 1:270–278, 1920

Seitz PFD: Psychocutaneous aspects of persistent pruritus and excessive excoriation. Arch Derm Syphilol 64:136–141, 1951

Simeon D, Stein DJ, Gross S, et al: A double-blind trial of fluoxetine in pathologic skin picking. J Clin Psychiatry 58:341–347, 1997

Stein DJ, Dodman NH, Borchelt P, et al: Behavioral disorders in veterinary practice: relevance to psychiatry. Compr Psychiatry 35:275–285, 1994

Stein DJ, Grant JE, Franklin ME, et al: Trichotillomania (hair-pulling disorder), skin picking disorder, and stereotypic movement disorder: toward DSM-V. Depress Anxiety 27:611–626, 2010

Stokes JH, Garner VC: The diagnosis of self-inflicted lesions of the skin. JAMA 93:438–443, 1929

Teng EJ, Woods DW, Twohig MP, et al: Body-focused repetitive behavior problems: prevalence in a nonreferred population and differences in perceived somatic activity. Behav Modif 26:340–360, 2002

Walther MR, Flessner CA, Conelea CA, et al: The Milwaukee Inventory for the Dimensions of Adult Skin Picking (MIDAS): initial development and psychometric properties. J Behav Ther Exp Psychiatry 40:127–135, 2009

Weintraub E, Robinson C, Newmeyer M: Catastrophic medical complication in psychogenic excoriation. South Med J 93:1099–1101, 2000

Wilhelm S, Keuthen NJ, Deckersbach T, et al: Self-injurious skin picking: clinical characteristics and comorbidity. J Clin Psychiatry 60:454–459, 1999

Wilson E: Lectures on Dermatology: Delivered in the Royal College of Surgeons of England, 1874–1875. London, J and A Churchill, 1875

Woods DW, Miltenberger RG, Flach AD: Habits, tics, and stuttering: prevalence and relation to anxiety and somatic awareness. Behav Modif 20:216–225, 1996

Woods DW, Flessner CA, Franklin ME, et al: The Trichotillomania Impact Project (TIP): exploring phenomenology, functional impairment, and treatment utilization. J Clin Psychiatry 67:1877–1888, 2006

Wrong NM: Excoriated acne of young females. Arch Derm Syphilol 70:576–582, 1954

Zaidens SH: Self-inflicted dermatoses and their psychodynamics. J Nerv Ment Disord 113:395–404, 1951

HABITUAL STEREOTYPIC MOVEMENTS

A Descriptive Analysis of Four Common Types

Greg Snyder, Ph.D.
Patrick C. Friman, Ph.D., ABPP

Motor stereotypies are defined as repetitive, habitual, non-goal-directed actions that are nonreflexive and under volitional control. Motor stereotypies are ubiquitous during the first year of life and rapidly begin dissipating by age 2 (Kravitz and Boehm 1971; Thelen 1979, 1981, 1996). The topography of any particular motor stereotypy can be as variable as any individual's behavioral repertoire. Most stereotypic movements, especially those frequently observed during infancy, are clinically benign. However, when these movements become grossly age-inappropriate, sufficiently disturbing, disruptive, or unhealthful, they are often classified as stereotypic movement disorder (SMD).

The progression from typical to atypical stereotypy involves, at its basic level, chronicity, resistance to intervention, and impairment. As an example, thumb sucking is universal and harmless in early infancy, whereas its chronic practice in the school-aged child can result in multiple threats to health, social standing, and psychological well-being (Friman and Schmitt 1989; Friman et al. 2006). Unfortunately, there is little research on functional classification of the various types of habitual stereotypical behavior, and the behaviors are typically grouped only according to topography. So a case involving fingernail biting may serve the functions more typically associated with SMD and yet be classified merely as fingernail biting. As another example, rhythmic head banging conducted as part of a sleep induction ritual is more appropriately classified with behaviors that serve the same purpose, such as thumb sucking or object attachment, but it is more likely to be classified as self-injurious head banging. Before the reader raises his or her hopes, we should point out that this chapter does not resolve this problem.

In this chapter, we define and describe four groups of stereotypic movement problems—thumb sucking, fingernail biting, SMD, and head banging—discussing prevalence, clinical characteristics, and prognoses. Because there are treatment literatures associated with all four, descriptions of treatments are confined to a few general comments and references to more thorough descriptions.

THUMB SUCKING

Definition

Sucking itself is an essential human activity that begins reflexively and continues because of the psychophysiological results it produces. Nonnutritional sucking, a virtually universal human activity in early life, occurs when children suck objects that are incapable of providing nutrition, such as fingers, toes, portions of the caregiver's body, or objects designed ad hoc, termed *pacifiers* in this culture and *dummies* in others (Friman et al. 2006). Although pacifier usage is common, *finger sucking* is by a wide margin the most commonly observed form of nonnutritional sucking. Finger sucking involves one readily observed core behavior (i.e., finger or fingers in mouth), and virtually all formal definitions include the operation of two lips touching or closing over at least one finger. Some definitions add topographical detail describing where the finger is placed (against the roof of the mouth) or the location of adjacent fingers (curled over the bridge of the nose or fisted with the other fingers). Lastly, some definitions include age and location criteria in order to distinguish potentially harmful from harmless finger sucking. For example, finger sucking can be considered chronic when it occurs in two or more social environments (e.g., home and school) after the age of 5 years (Friman 2003a; Friman and Schmitt 1989).

Epidemiology

As indicated, finger sucking is almost universal in infancy. In neonates, estimated rates of finger sucking reach as high as 95%. In fact, finger sucking is so prevalent in newborns that its absence is sometimes interpreted as a risk factor for physical or developmental problems. For example, the absence of healthy sucking during infancy can be indicative of feeding problems, and research has shown significant associations between early infant feeding/ sucking difficulties and failure to thrive and growth deficiencies (Emond et al. 2007). The absence of strong, rapid sucking in neonates is associated with neurological dysfunction and later developmental delay (Medoff-Cooper et al. 2009). Because of its reflexive onset, almost universal early presence, and potential development benefits, finger sucking is not typically even discussed as a problematic habit until the toddler years.

Estimates of problematic finger sucking vary, but generally decline as children age and develop, with prevalence estimates of 50% of children at ages 2–3 years (Infante 1976; Klackenberg 1949; Ozturk and Ozturk 1977; Popovich and Thompson 1974), declining to approximately 25% of 5-year-olds (Klackenberg 1949; Mahalski and Stanton 1992). Variable estimates of the prevalence of finger sucking are also present in older children, ranging from 11% at 11 years of age to as high as 28% (Mahalski and Stanton 1992; Popovich and Thompson 1974).

Clinical Characteristics

Finger sucking is healthful or at least harmless for very young children, but continued practice beyond the age of 4 or 5 years increasingly places the children at risk physically and psychologically. The most common physical risk involves problematic formation of teeth. Chronic sucking can have an effect on emerging teeth and bite formation (e.g., malocclusion) and can necessitate extensive (and expensive) orthodontic intervention for repair (Friman and Schmitt 1989; Leung and Robson 1990; Warren et al. 2001). Intense sucking of the thumb or finger creates pressure imbalances between the teeth, tongue, and hard and soft palates, resulting in anterior misalignment, overbite, and crossbite. Risk for crossbite in chronic thumb-sucking children is three times that in the normal population (Peterson 1982). Children with chronic thumb sucking are also at increased risk for abnormal facial growth (Moore et al. 1972), digital deformities (Campbell-Reid and Prince 1984; Rankin et al. 1988), recurrent skin infections (Vogel 1998), and accidental poisonings (Turbeville and Fearnow 1976). There are psychological risks as well, the most common of which involves adverse social reaction and even rejection. A study of thumb sucking in first-grade children showed that those who sucked fingers were viewed as less attractive and intelligent and less preferred as seatmates, classmates, neighbors, and friends than nonsucking peers (Friman et al. 1993). Other psychological risks include problematic interactions with parents.

Finger sucking is also often correlated with other self-soothing behaviors such as attachment to a "transitional object," with estimates of thumb-sucking children who habitually carry such objects ranging as high as 50% (Mahalski

1983). Such objects have also been shown to increase the motivation to suck (Friman 2000), and their removal has been shown to be an effective means of reducing or eliminating sucking (e.g., Friman 1990). Although the object attachment associated with thumb sucking is almost always benign, sucking does co-occur with other stereotypical behaviors that are not, the best example of which is chronic hair pulling. There are no epidemiological studies on the prevalence of co-occurring finger sucking and hair pulling, but there are multiple case descriptions in the treatment literature (e.g., Friman and Hove 1987).

A concern about finger sucking, persistent from Freud forward to the present day, involves the belief that its practice reflects underlying psychopathology. A substantial and growing body of research has dismissed this concern, however, for all but a very tiny minority of finger-sucking children (e.g., Friman et al. 1994, 2006). Additionally, the extensive number and problematic nature of problems in this minority usually render sucking a secondary concern.

One important question left virtually unanswered by research is what causes extended thumb sucking. The small body of existing research demonstrating the influence of attachment objects on the initiation and maintenance of thumb sucking represents the only effort, thus far, to experimentally determine causal variables associated with the persistence of this behavior. Although clinical and anecdotal reports of increased frequency during periods of fatigue, boredom, anxiety, or anger are abundant, no actual experimental research has been conducted to determine the presence and strength of any such relationship. Research has shown that finger sucking produces a psychophysiological effect, reduced arousal (e.g., self-soothing, comforting). A large body of scientific evidence has demonstrated this effect, especially in very young children, and most adults have witnessed the effect in vivo by watching crying children seek comfort from their thumb or finger or calm quickly when given a pacifier (Friman et al. 2006). It seems plausible, if not self-evident, that this effect is potentially habit-forming. So, although not yet scientifically verified, it appears likely that extended thumb sucking is maintained in either of two ways: positive reinforcement produced by the pleasure of the act or negative reinforcement produced by relief obtained from the act. Very early in life, the procurement of pleasure and relief via sucking is normal and expected, but chronic practice beyond the age of 4 or 5 years may suggest a deficiency in more mature methods of procuring these psychological outcomes.

Prognosis

Finger sucking in children is virtually nonexistent by the time children reach 14 years of age, and for those who persist in the behavior, it occurs so privately and infrequently that the risk for harm is negligible. Additionally, any problems caused by the sucking, even in chronic cases, have also usually been remediated by then. However, although we found no research on thumb sucking in adulthood, evidence that the habit continues into the adult years is abundant. Its prevalence and prognosis (i.e., is thumb sucking in adulthood as benign as suggested?) are not possible to determine, at least not with the level of assurance required by typical readers of this book. Presently, the only available sources of information on adult thumb sucking are in media or on the Internet. For a glimpse of the phenomena, merely type "adult thumb sucking" into a search window on a favorite browser (e.g., Google, Bing) and view some of the top sites that are listed.

NAIL BITING

Definition

Nail biting (onychophagia) is the term for repetitive biting and/or chewing of the fingernails (and sometimes toenails) (Friman 2003b). Early research based on covert observations indicated that the following steps compose the act of nail biting: 1) placing the hand near the mouth; 2) placing the finger against the teeth; 3) beginning biting and chewing; and 4) withdrawing the finger and inspecting the nail(s) bitten (Billig 1941). As with other oral habits such as thumb sucking, nail biting was once thought to be part of a constellation of symptoms suggestive of serious underlying psychopathology but is now merely classified as a simple habit when its practice has not led to unhealthful consequences (e.g., cuticle damage, social problems) and a habit disorder when it has. Although the literature on treatment of nail biting is substantial and reasonably rigorous (e.g., Allen 1996; Azrin et al. 1980), the research pertinent to the discussion in this chapter is limited in many ways, and thus our treatment of it will be brief. For example, clear operational definitions that supply topographical, frequency, and age criteria either are not used or are typically not reported. A stark exception insofar as topography is concerned is found in Billig (1941), whose definition we used previously. The thoroughness and clarity of Billig's topographical description has not only not been improved upon in the research to follow—it has not even been matched.

Epidemiology

The limited availability of operational definitions reduces the utility of, or at least confidence in, reports on the prevalence of nail biting. Furthermore, the prevalence data that are reported are often inconsistent. For example, an early study reported that 44% of children at age 13 were nail biters (Wechsler 1931), and a later study reported a prevalence of only 12% in a similar age group (Deardoff et al. 1974). The literature is also often highly derivative, with more current papers typically relying on earlier studies that supplied neither operational definitions nor information on research methods. For example, the figures supplied by Wechsler (1931) are central to an early review by Massler and Malone (1950) that is, in turn, central to a current review by Leung and Robson (1990). Additionally, some papers offer prevalence figures without supplying supportive citations (e.g., Peterson 1982). One study (Malone and Massler 1952), however, stands out from the rest in terms of its sample size (N=4,587, ages 5–18 years), definitions (varied based on degree of nail biting), and methods (direct interview and observation of the participants' fingernails). Nonetheless, this study is dated. Another study, also dated, stands out in terms of its sample size (N=6,946) but not in terms of the definitional criteria for establishing the presence or absence of biting. Its data support the estimates provided below and extend the analysis to age 37 years (Pennington 1945). There are two more recent studies, but their focus extends to nervous habits in general and only in younger children (Foster 1998; Troster 1994). Having offered those caveats, we here present our best guess at onset and prevalence.

Nail biting is rarely observed before age 3. Prevalence rates generally increase between the ages of 4 and 6, remain level between 7 and 10, and rise again and peak at the onset of adolescence (i.e., puberty), with estimates ranging from 25% to 60%. Prevalence then declines through the adolescent years, with estimates between 20% and 30% for the late teens. Prevalence in young adults ranges between 10% and 25% and declines to below 10% for adults over 35.

The literature on gender is also inconsistent; some studies report a higher prevalence among females (DeFrancesco et al. 1989; Hadley 1984), whereas others report a higher prevalence in males (Birch 1955; Coleman and McCalley 1948; Joubert 1993). The safest conclusion we can draw here is that nail biting appears to be a common habit across genders (but current, reliable quantitative specifics are unavailable).

Clinical Characteristics

Surprisingly, and in contrast with other dimensions of their respective literatures, we found more empirically derived information on the clinical characteristics of nail biting than we did on finger sucking. The literature indicates that nail biting is typically confined to the fingernails but can involve toenails (Leung and Robson 1990). Malone and Massler (1952), in their study, showed that nail biters show little preference toward any of their fingers in particular. The Billig (1941) study that provided the description used in our definition was conducted covertly, and not only did it yield a clear picture of the sequence of steps in the act of nail biting (i.e., hand near the mouth, finger against the teeth, biting, chewing, withdrawal, and inspection), it also showed that nail biting is highly responsive to audience variables; the participants in the Billig study immediately ceased the practice when they were observed.

Beyond a single report that nail biting occurs more frequently in monozygotic versus dyzygotic twins (Bakwin 1971), thus suggesting a genetic etiology, there is no available research directly related to cause. Multiple papers, however, have correlated nail biting with a broad range of exotic psychological variables, such as sociopathy (Walker and Ziskind 1977), hostility (Coleman 1950), bipolarity (Endicott 1989), and suicide risk (Weinlander and Lee 1978). A less exotic and more frequently reported association involves anxiety or stress, but the supportive literature suffers from the types of contradictions and derivative problems that plague the literature on prevalence. For example, two early and influential papers asserted a relationship between nail biting and anxiety (or tension), but experimental control subjects were not employed in the research described, nor were persuasive data presented (e.g., Massler and Malone 1950; Wechsler 1931). Nonetheless, a later review reported that the relationship between nail biting and anxiety is well documented and cited the two papers as supportive evidence (Leung and Robson 1990).

Confusing matters further are other papers that appear to refute the relationship (e.g., Deardoff et al. 1974; Joubert 1993), with still others that appear to support it. Prominent among the supportive studies are two demonstrating that "nervous habits" such as nail biting may indeed be associated with increases in anxiety (Woods and Miltenberger 1996; Woods et al. 1996). However, in neither study was nail biting isolated from the other habits studied to determine whether it had independent functions.

A few studies suggest that nail biting in older youth and young adults may have a detrimental effect on self-evaluation and social functioning. For example, college students who bit their nails were reported to perceive their appearance and health more negatively than persons who did not bite their nails (Hansen et al. 1990). Related (albeit less rigorous) research reported that adult nail biters are at risk for feeling shameful, experiencing low self-esteem, exhibiting social avoidance, and suffering occupational impairment (Joubert 1993). These internalizing associations may (when present) be at least partly due to social consequences. Nail biters can be the victims of negative social perceptions by others because the habit is often believed to be associated with multiple types of disturbance, such as inattention, deficient social skills, and nervousness. In addition, some (perhaps many) persons perceive nail biting as a socially unacceptable, undesirable, and repulsive habit (Silber and Haynes 1992; Wells et al. 1998).

Some associations involving medical complications have also been documented. For example, nail biting can damage the cuticle, nail, and skin surface of the fingertip (Leung and Robson 1990). Habitual biting can increase nail growth by as much as 20% (Bean 1980). As with finger sucking, secondary bacterial infection, especially of the cuticle, can result from nail biting (Baron and Dawber 1984). The emergence of periungual warts has also been documented (Samman 1977). Lastly, like finger sucking, chronic nail biting can inhibit oral hygiene and impair dentition (e.g., atypical root absorption; Odenrick and Brattstrom 1985).

Prognosis

As contrasted with thumb sucking, the literature on nail biting does include data on the extent of the habit into the adult years (e.g., Pennington 1945), with estimates of 8%–10%. Unfortunately, there are no data on the well-being of adult-aged nail biters. However, whereas adult-aged thumb suckers are readily capable of practicing their habit covertly, thus avoiding social stigma, and temperately, thus avoiding physical harm, adult-aged nail biters may be more susceptible to social costs and physical problems. Regarding social costs, although it is possible to hide the act of nail biting, it can be hard to hide its cosmetically and medically damaging effects (e.g., Iorizzo et al. 2007). The act of nail biting itself involves damaging part of the body, with the potential extent of the damage discussed earlier. Although nail biting is not clearly correlated with psychological problems, the widespread assumption that its practice suggests something potentially stigmatizing or unflattering about its practitioner could become a self-fulfilling prophecy due to social reaction. This is merely reasonably well-informed speculation, however, because of the gaps in the literature. The extant data do show that nail biting is associated with multiple physical side effects and that its practice diminishes with age. What that practice does to practitioners who continue on into their adult years is presently unknown.

RHYTHMIC/STEREOTYPIC MOVEMENTS AND STEREOTYPIC MOVEMENT DISORDER

Definition

As stated in the introduction to this chapter, rhythmic and/or stereotypic behavior and SMD differ in chronicity, resistance to intervention, and impairment. SMD represents a diagnostic classification of motor behavior that is "repetitive, often seemingly driven, and nonfunctional" (DSM-IV-TR; American Psychiatric Association 2000) and either results in injury or significantly interferes with the routine activities of daily child life. Historically, studies examining the prevalence and developmental trajectories of stereotypic behavior have involved separate investigations of typically developing children on one hand and those with developmental disturbances on the other. Of the available studies that have examined SMD, often in the context of other neurological or neurodevelopmental issues, operationalized definitions that discriminate between rhythmic, stereotyped behavior and SMD are absent, limiting in-depth knowledge about underlying differences or similarities between these classes of behaviors. Of the studies that have attempted classification of stereotypic behaviors, the methods employed often conflict, making it difficult to aggregate data meaningfully across studies. These inconsistencies have also made it challenging to create a decision-making framework, other than one relying on clinical intuition, for defining SMD beyond typically emergent stereotypic behavior patterns.

Initial interest in stereotypic movement can be found in the developmental literature. Early naturalistic observations of infants described the phenomena, "rhythmic motor movements," as repeated, non-goal-directed motor actions exhibited by virtually all infants during their first year of life. Psychiatry, neurology, and other medical disciplines have traditionally used terminology such as *stereotypic behavior* or *stereotypies* to describe the movements when they persist, although the age when such a distinction is made is usually based on clinical judgment. The lack of consensus on the technical term used to describe both normal and abnormal variations of these movements has resulted in poor definitional consistency and, at times, conflicting findings on the natural course and differentiation between normal and abnormal stereotypic behavior. The limitations in the relevant literature notwithstanding, the following paragraphs include our best efforts at describing/defining stereotypic motor movements.

Benign stereotypic motor behavior presenting universally during infant development has been methodically described and categorized during the past quarter century. Thelen (1979) originally organized rhythmic motor movements by the parts of the body used in the movements, such as rhythmic kicking (alternate legs, single leg kicks, and foot rubbing), torso movements (e.g., rocking, posturing, swaying, and bouncing), arm/hand movements (e.g., waving, flexion/extension of the hands, clapping), and head motions (e.g., head rolling, nodding, shaking). Subsequent efforts to document benign stereotypic motor behavior have typically used these early descriptions.

Clinically significant stereotypic motor movement, or SMD, is generally considered to be an extreme variant of benign stereotypies and is parsed into two broad categories based upon the presence or absence of other neurological findings (Mahone et al. 2004): pathological and physiological. *Pathological stereotypic movements* are often seen in persons with preexisting sensory conditions (i.e., blindness and deafness), mental retardation, autism, infection, tumor, or other psychiatric illness (Mahone et al. 2004; Muthogovindan and Singer 2009). *Physiological stereotypic movements* are not associated with preexisting conditions and are subdivided according to body parts involved in the movements observed. Alternative categorizations have been offered by psychiatry and neurology and include 1) common motor stereotypies (body rocking, head banging, thumb sucking, nail biting, and hair twirling), 2) head nodding/rolling, and 3) complex motor behaviors (hand shaking, flapping, waving, finger writhing, arm flapping, and flexion/extension of the hands and wrists) (Muthugovindan and Singer 2009). Given the substantial differences in definition and categorization, comparison across studies is problematic.

Epidemiology

Developmentally, the emergence of motor stereotypies often coincides with increased volitional control of separate motor systems, leading some theorists to speculate that these early repetitive, rhythmic behaviors reflect an immature and incomplete stage of motor development (Thelen 1979, 1981). As noted in the beginning of the chapter, a wide range of stereotypic movements, such as toe and finger/hand/thumb sucking, foot kicking, body rocking, head banging, and arm waving, occur in a vast majority of infants during the first 2 years of life (Thelen 1979, 1981, 1996). Kravits and Boehm (1971) observed that hand writhing, lip sucking/biting, and body rocking were present in more that 90% of the infants studied, with all rhythmic movements emerging before age 2 in typically developing infants. Head rolling and head banging were less frequently observed (20% and 7%, respectively) and emerged later than other stereotypic movements (average age >12 months). Kravits and Boehm (1971) also reported increased prevalence of rhythmic behavior in boys compared with girls (3.5:1). Infants with intellectual disabilities and Down syndrome were indistinguishable from normal infants in terms of the frequency of stereotypic or rhythmic movements, but their movements were distinguished by a delayed onset.

Similar to early observations of typically developing and at-risk infants, Werry et al. (1983) reported that thumb/finger sucking, pacifier use, and head banging emerged before 24 months in 75% of infants studied. Thumb/finger sucking was virtually ubiquitous during the first 3–5 months of life, with a deceleration in the rate of thumb/finger sucking to 19% by age 5. Consistent with earlier observations (e.g., Kravitz and Boehm 1971), the emergence and peak incidence of head banging occurred later than other stereotypic movements, peaking at 20% at 12–17 months of age but rapidly declining to 0.3% at age 5. Throughout the entire sample, virtually all stereotypic behaviors had disappeared by age 5 (Werry et al. 1983).

Troster (1994) provided data on 142 typically developing children between 10 months and 11 years of age who were living in residential care. More than half (58.5%) of the entire sample exhibited at least one motor stereotypy per week, with nearly one-quarter exhibiting at least one stereotypic behavior per day. Forty percent of the children studied exhibited stereotyped movements multiple times per day, with nearly 30% displaying more than one category of stereotypy. Although the study recorded high frequency of stereotypic behavior overall, the number of cases and the frequency of movements declined with age. During infancy and toddlerhood, thumb sucking, hair twisting, and body rocking were the most frequent, transitioning to nail biting and finger chewing/mouthing for children in the oldest subset, ages 6–11. Similarly, Leekam et al. (2007) summarized parent/caregiver reports of stereotypic movements and indicated that 20% of children exhibited repetitive hand and/or finger movements one or more times per day, with nearly 10% emitting these behaviors 15 or more times per day. The authors also reported body rocking in 18% of the study population one or more times per day. A much smaller percentage of the children (2%) exhibited body rocking 15 or more times per day.

As suggested earlier, typically developing children almost universally exhibit stereotypic behavior, with a steep linear decline in frequency and virtual disappearance by age 5. Children with intellectual delays also exhibit stereotypic behavior, but its timing, trajectory, and quality of movement differ substantively from those of the stereotypy exhibited by typically developing children. The stereotypy of children with delays begins later in life and tends to last much longer. More importantly, the stereotypy of children with delays has a much greater risk of creating impairment and thus becoming clinically significant (e.g., Hall et al. 2001, 2003).

In an attempt to clarify the often subjective differences between "normal" rhythmic behavior and "atypical" stereotypy among children with and without developmental delays, Schwartz et al. (1986) observed increased amplitude and frequency of body rocking among infants with intellectual delays as compared with typically developing children. MacLean et al. (1991) compared matched (on Bayley Developmental Motor Age scores; Bayley 1969) nondisabled, Down syndrome, and motor-impaired children on the presence and variability of normal rhythmic activity. Even when motor age was roughly controlled for, Down syndrome and motor-impaired children displayed slower emergence of age-typical stereotypic motor behavior. Moreover, the stereotypic movements exhibited in the developmentally delayed children were qualitatively different than movements exhibited by the typically developing children (i.e., increased rates of rhythmic mouth and foot movements). Wehmeyer (1991, 1994) examined children at risk for moderate, severe, and profound mental retardation and also reported delayed onset of age-typical stereotypic motor behavior. Similar to MacLean et al. (1991), Wehmeyer noted increased frequency of "atypical" stereotyped or rhythmic motor behavior.

Evidence for qualitative distinctions in the rhythmic motor activity exhibited by individuals with developmental delays has also been observed in children with genetic disorders, such as cri du chat syndrome (a chromosomal disorder featuring a distinctive facial appearance, growth retardation, microcephaly, delayed development, moderate to severe intellectual disability, and minimal to no speech). In one notable study, nearly 60% of the children and adolescents observed displayed two or more stereotypic behaviors simultaneously, with a large majority exhibiting rhythmic, stereotyped behavior (86%) that was potentially self-injurious (head banging, vomiting, biting, bruxism, and skin picking/scratching being most frequently reported; Collins and Cornish 2002).

Among children with autism and autism spectrum disorders (ASDs), rhythmic, stereotyped behavior also appears to be more frequent and qualitatively different from that exhibited by typically developing children. Richler et al. (2007) observed increased rates of stereotypic hand/finger movements and complex mannerisms among children with ASD and ASD with concurrent developmental delays as compared with typically developing children (53.7% and 61.6% vs. 9.2%). Differences in the frequency of stereotypic behavior were also noticeable when comparing developmentally delayed children who had an ASD with developmentally delayed children who did not. The children who had ASD exhibited more types and higher frequencies of stereotypic motor movements (20.4% and 18.4%, respectively).

Findings from other recent research replicate the findings of Richler et al. (2007) suggesting significant differences in the onset and trajectory of rhythmic, stereotypic movements between typically developing children and children with ASD or other developmental delays. For example, in a study involving direct observation of delayed children with and without ASD, Goldman et al. (2008) reported that nearly half of the children studied exhibited at least one stereotypy but that the initial onset was later in children with ASD. The children with ASD also exhibited more stereotypical behaviors. Thus, the co-occurrence of ASD and developmental delay appeared to exert a compounding effect in terms of chronicity and frequency of stereotypic motor behavior. Stereotypic behavior emerges in typically developing persons with psychiatric conditions at about the same time it does in typically developing persons without such conditions, but it appears to be more persistent in the former group. For example, in a study of 40 clinic-referred children presenting with stereotypic movement (25% with attention-deficit/hyperactivity disorder, 18% with tic disorder, 20% with learning disabilities, 5% with obsessive-compulsive disorder [OCD]), only 5% had ceased their stereotypic movement by age 12 years, a substantial departure from 5 years, the age at which virtually all typically developing children have ceased exhibition of stereotypy.

To summarize, despite multiple attempts at using behavioral topography to distinguish types of stereotypy in persons with and without intellectual disabilities or psychiatric disturbance, the only distinctive features appear to involve onset, persistence, and differential severity. It appears that all human infants exhibit a wide range of rhythmic, stereotyped motor movements early in life, with deceleration and disappearance of the movements in typically developing children by 24–60 months of age. In typically developing children, the movements rarely become severe enough to warrant the label of SMD. The timing of the transition of "normal" rhythmic motor behavior to "abnormal" stereotypy or SMD is ill-defined at present, but the transition appears to occur after age 5 years. In persons with developmental delays, stereotyped motor movements emerge later in life, persist longer, are exhibited with more frequency and intensity, and are at heightened risk for devolving into SMD. In persons who begin life with typical development but subsequently develop a significant psychiatric condition, stereotypy has an early onset but a differential persistence and quality and is also at heightened risk for devolving to SMD. Thus, although the causal pathway is not clear, some combination of delayed onset, persistence, and differential quality of presentation likely contributes to the increased risk for SMD in impaired persons.

Clinical Characteristics

Rhythmic or stereotypic behaviors can resemble behaviors associated with serious neurological and psychiatric conditions such as OCD, Tourette syndrome, chronic tic disorder, chorea, athetosis, muscle dystonia, and tardive dyskinesia. An informed clinical assessment, however, can readily rule out these serious conditions. For example, SMD is readily distinguished from OCD and tics/Tourette syndrome through the absence of mounting internal "urges" in SMD. Additionally, stereotypic behavior is easily interrupted without a buildup of internal tension or internal emotional distress. As another example, the repetitive behaviors observed in OCD are ritualized, complex behaviors and/or thoughts that function to avoid or minimize anxiety or emotional distress. Abrupt cessation of the ritual is associated with significant distress and impairment, which is not the case with the movements seen in SMD. Furthermore, gradual voluntary suppression is not associated with increased tension or stress, as it is in Tourette syndrome. Stereotypic movements and SMD are also differentiated from chorea (rapid jerking that may or may not be incorporated into voluntary movement), athetosis (slowed writhing movements), muscle dystonia (postural disturbances created through simultaneous contraction of agonist and antagonist muscle groups), and tardive dyskinesia (often involving buccolingual masticatory movements), because those afflicted with these conditions often cannot control the symptomatic behaviors volitionally, whereas persons afflicted with SMD can. Additionally, the symptomatic behaviors in the neurological conditions often occur during sleep, whereas the symptomatic behaviors in SMD rarely do (Fenichel 1997).

Prognosis

Stereotypic movements are common and universal among typically developing infants, usually resolving without specific treatment or intervention. Stereotypic behaviors involving the hands and mouth (i.e., finger/thumb sucking, pacifier use), extremities (e.g., hand/arm waving, rhythmic leg movements), or body/trunk broadly appear within the first year of life and disappear as the infant gains strength and volitional control of the motor system. As a result, these behaviors diminish during the second and third year of life, and most disappear by age 4–5 years. Thus when the movements are present in children without intellectual delay, the likelihood that clinical attention is warranted is quite low. Furthermore, in cases in which treatment is required, it would likely be brief, involving only consultation, psychoeducation, and/or basic management. However, the stereotypic movements exhibited by persons with psychiatric disturbance, intellectual delay, or neurodevelopmental disorder appear to be more frequent, intense, and resistant to treatment. Thus the prognosis in impaired populations is more guarded and the treatments needed more intensive.

HEAD BANGING

Definition

Head banging involves a constellation of behaviors whose apparent purpose is either to bring the head into contact with fixed objects (e.g., floor, wall) or to purposely strike the head with hands or objects. In contemporary colloquial use, the term *head banging* has come to denote vigorous flexion and extension of the neck to music, most often heavy metal/hard rock music (Jackson et al. 1983), and not banging of the head against either fixed or movable objects. However, this definition is well beyond the current scope of this chapter, and this action has never been characterized as a stereotypic movement. As suggested earlier, head banging numbers among the more commonly observed motor stereotypies appearing during infancy. In an early observational analysis of head banging during infancy, De Lissovoy (1963) described four variants organized along the position and posturing of the child during the behavior: 1) positioned on all fours, striking the top of the head against a fixed object; 2) positioned supine, striking typically the posterior region of the head against the ground; 3) seated upright, striking the head against a fixed object; and 4) lying prone, striking the anterior of the head. A fifth orientation was described simply as a combination of these postures and positions. When occurring in typically developing infants and children, head banging is most frequently observed before normal sleep (De Lissovoy 1963; Leung and Robson 1990).

Epidemiology

When appearing as a part of normal infant motor development, head banging appears to develop later than other rhythmic motor behavior, ranging from 8.6 months to 1 year, with cessation typically by age 4 (Kravitz and Boehm 1971; Sallustro and Atwell 1978), although two studies have reported persistence for a very small number of children past age 10 (De Lissovoy 1963; Hashizume et al. 2002). Unlike the ubiquitous nature of other stereotypic movements, such as thumb/finger sucking, body rocking, and arm waving, head banging occurs less frequently in typically developing children, with prevalence estimates ranging from 3.3% to 15.2% (Kravitz and Boehm 1971; Sallustro and Atwell 1978; Thelen 1979, 1981). Sallustro and Atwell (1978) reported that head banging occurred in 5.1% of a sample of 525 healthy, typically developing children, with increased rates of head banging among boys over girls (3:1). These estimates are similar to those provided by Kravitz and Boehm (1971).

Clinical Characteristics

Of all stereotypic behaviors that have been systematically evaluated, head banging occurs much less frequently among typically developing children and has a much shorter course. Thus, the risk for injury is low when the infant or child experiences and responds to naturally occurring contingencies associated with the behavior (i.e., pain). Although viewed as normal and generally harmless among typically developing infants and children, head banging in persons with intellectual delay or neurodevelopmental disorder is at increased risk for escalation and persistence, possibly because of operant processes (e.g., Iwata et al. 1994). Head banging, especially when intractable and severe, is associated with a number of medically significant complications. In fact, both acute and cumulative trauma to the head as a result of self-injurious stereotypic head banging are not unlike the long-term consequences of contact sports such as boxing and football. Chronic subdural hematomas, retinal hemorrhages and detachment, cataracts, encephalopathy, enlarged ventricles, and dental injuries are some of the serious long-term consequences of untreated, sustained head banging (Spalter et al. 1970).

A clear negative correlation between the frequency and intensity of self-injurious head banging and intellectual ability has been documented, with lower IQ placing individuals at increased risk for severe and persistent head banging (Berkson 1983). Self-injurious head banging is more common in those children with intellectual impairments and associated developmental disorders, including autism (e.g., Adrien et al. 1987; Bodfish et al. 2000; Dawson et al. 2000; Nijhof et al. 1998), cri du chat syndrome, Rett syndrome, Cornelia de Lange syndrome, and Prader-Willi syndrome (Dykens and Kasari 1997; Symons et al. 2003). Robey et al. (2003) reported head banging as the second most frequent form of self-injurious behavior in children with Lesch-Nyhan syndrome (rare, X-linked recessive chromosomal disorder). Collins and Cornish (2002), in a study of children with cri du chat syndrome, reported moderate to severe head banging in nearly half of all affected subjects evaluated, along with other serious self-injurious behavior such as self-biting, scratching, bruxism, and hair pulling.

Prognosis

In early published observations of head banging in children, onset was described as ritualized, habit-like behavior that immediately preceded sleep onset, similar to thumb sucking or pacifier use. Multiple studies of head banging in typically developing children suggest it occurs much less frequently than other stereotypic movements and usually subsides without treatment. Among typically developing infants and children, head banging poses little risk of harm. Head banging alone is not associated with a concurrent or future risk for psychopathology or cognitive delay, despite the fact that persons with cognitive delays exhibit increased rates and a more problematic course (Abe et al. 1984). Sallustro and Atwell (1978) studied multiple dimensions of development in typically developing children and found that head-banging children differed on only two: 1) age the child first held his or her head erect, and 2) age the child first walked without support. Similar results were reported by Abe et al. (1984) in a 5-year follow-up study of 3-year-old children exhibiting head banging, head rolling, and breath holding, none of which predicted future disturbance of cognitive functioning or behavior. Contrasted with the brief duration of head banging in typically developing children, head banging in persons with intellectual delays is usually much more persistent; it is also much more strongly associated with bodily harm and it requires much more intensive behavioral/environmental modifications for successful remediation.

CONCLUSION

We described four common types of habitual stereotyped movements, with special emphasis on definition, epidemiology, clinical characteristics, and prognosis. Although we would like to claim that the review in this chapter significantly extends the literature, modesty bids that we claim merely that we collated extant information well. From the information we gathered, at least three suggestions for further study present themselves. First and most importantly, although functional analysis has been available since the early 1970s, stereotyped movements are still classified mostly according to topography. Thus, as briefly discussed earlier in the chapter, mild, sleep-inducting head banging in an infant could be captured in the same epidemiological class as self-injurious head banging in an adult with developmental disabilities. Analyzing both types according to their respective functions would almost certainly result in distinct classifications.

Another suggestion involves further study of the importance of age at onset. In typically developing children, stereotypic movements are virtually universal in infancy, then dissipate steadily and, with the exception of fingernail biting and thumb sucking, virtually disappear by school age. However, in persons with developmental disabilities, these movements emerge later in life and remain much longer. Needed are descriptive and experimental analyses to determine whether stereotyped movements in these persons are delayed merely as a function of the overall developmental delay or because they represent a different type of behavior altogether.

Finally, because of the bizarre topography of many stereotypic movements and the seeming meaninglessness of most, persons who exhibit them are at risk for being classified according to some dimension of psychopathology. Needed is research that addresses the question of psychopathology in children exhibiting stereotypy as it has been addressed in children exhibiting other problematic behavior (e.g., Friman 2002; Friman et al. 1988, 1994, 1998). Although the influence of the dynamic model (and its attendant use of psychopathology as an explanatory mechanism) is on the wane, it still emerges in the movement literature from time to time and is also still very much alive in the lay community. Therefore, new research identifying more parsimonious, empirically verifiable causal mechanisms is needed. In closing, not all movements have a purpose. Yet the absence of purpose in the presence of movement does not also mean the presence of illness or defect. What it does mean, however, is still not entirely clear. New research, especially that focused on function, could make things more clear.

REFERENCES

Abe K, Oda N, Amatomi M: Natural history and predictive significance of head-banging, head-rolling, and breath-holding spells. Dev Med Child Neurol 26:644–648, 1984

Adrien JL, Ornitz EM, Barthelemy C, et al: The presence or absence of certain behaviors associated with infantile autism in severely retarded autistic and non-autistic retarded children and very young normal children. J Autism Dev Disord 17:407–416, 1987

Allen KW: Chronic nailbiting: a controlled comparison of competing response and mild aversion treatments. Behav Res Ther 34:269–272, 1996

American Psychiatric Association: Diagnostic and Statistical Manual of Mental Disorders, 4th Edition, Text Revision. Washington, DC, American Psychiatric Association, 2000

Azrin N, Nunn RG, Frantz SE: Habit reversal vs. negative practice treatment of nail biting. Behav Res Ther 18:281–285, 1980

Bakwin H: Nail-biting in twins. Dev Med Child Neurol 13:304–307, 1971

Baron R, Dawber RPR: Diseases of the Nails and Their Management. Oxford, United Kingdom, Blackwell Scientific, 1984

Bayley N: Bayley Scales of Infant Development. New York, The Psychological Corporation, 1969

Bean WB: Nail growth: thirty five years of observation. Arch Intern Med 140:73–76, 1980

Berkson G: Repetitive sterotypical behaviors. Am J Ment Defic 88:239–246, 1983

Billig AL: Fingernail biting: its incipiency, incidence, and amelioration. Genetic Psychological Monographs 24:123–218, 1941

Birch LB: The incidence of nail biting among school children. Br J Educ Psychol 25:123–128, 1955

Bodfish JW, Symons FJ, Parker DE, et al: Varieties of repetitive behavior in autism: comparisons to mental retardation. J Autism Dev Disord 30:237–243, 2000

Campbell-Reid D, Price A: Digital deformities and dental malocclusion due to finger sucking. Br J Plast Surg 37:445–452, 1984

Coleman JC: The role of hostility in fingernail biting. Psychological Service Center Journal 3:238–244, 1950

Coleman JC, McCalley JE: Nail biting among college students. J Abnorm Soc Psychol 43:517–525, 1948

Collins MSR, Cornish K: A survey of the prevalence of stereotypy, self-injury and aggression in children and young adults with Cri du Chat syndrome. J Intellect Disabil Res 46:133–140, 2002

Dawson G, Osterling J, Meltzoff A, et al: Case study of the development of an infant with autism from birth to two years of age. J Appl Dev Psychol 21:299–313, 2000

Deardoff PA, Finch AJ Jr, Royall LR: Manifest anxiety and nail-biting. J Clin Psychol 30:378, 1974

DeFrancesco JJ, Zahner GEP, Pawelkiewicz W: Childhood nail biting. J Soc Behav Pers 4:157–161, 1989

De Lissovoy V: Head banging in early childhood. Child Dev 33:43–56, 1963

Dykens EM, Kasari C: Maladaptive behavior in children with Prader-Willi syndrome, Down syndrome, and nonspecific mental retardation. Am J Ment Retard 102:228–237, 1997

Emond A, Drewett R, Blair P, et al: Postnatal factors associated with failure to thrive in term infants in the Avon Longitudinal Study of Parents and Children. Arch Dis Child 92:115–119, 2007

Endicott NA: Psychophysiological correlates of 'bipolarity.' J Affect Disord 17:47–56, 1989

Fenichel GM: Movement disorders, in Clinical Pediatric Neurology: A Signs and Symptoms Approach. Philadelphia, PA, WB Saunders/Harcourt Brace, 1997, pp 292–309

Foster LG: Nervous habits and stereotyped behaviors in preschool children. J Am Acad Child Adolesc Psychiatry 37:711–717, 1998

Friman PC: Concurrent habits: what would Linus do with his blanket if his thumb-sucking were treated? Am J Dis Child 144:1316–1318, 1990

Friman PC: 'Transitional objects' as establishing operations for thumb sucking: a case study. J Appl Behav Anal 34:507–509, 2000

Friman PC: The psychopathological interpretation of common child behavior problems: a critique and related opportunity for behavior analysis. Invited address at the 28th annual convention of the Association for Behavior Analysis, Toronto, Canada, May 2002

Friman PC: Finger sucking, in Encyclopedia of Pediatric and Child Psychology. Edited by Ollendick T, Schroeder C. New York, Kluwer, 2003a, pp 238–240

Friman PC: Nail biting, in Encyclopedia of Pediatric and Child Psychology. Edited by Ollendick T, Schroeder C. New York, Kluwer, 2003b, pp 394–395

Friman PC, Hove G: Apparent covariation between child habit disorders: effects of successful treatment for thumb sucking on untargeted chronic hair pulling. J Appl Behav Anal 20:421–426, 1987

Friman PC, Schmitt BD: Thumb sucking: guidelines for pediatricians. Clin Pediatr 28:438–440, 1989

Friman PC, Mathews J, Finney JW, et al: Do encopretic children have clinically significant behavior problems? Pediatrics 82:407–409, 1988

Friman PC, McPherson KM, Warzak WJ, et al: The influence of chronic thumb sucking on peer social acceptance in first-grade children. Pediatrics 91:784–786, 1993

Friman PC, Larzelere R, Finney JW: Exploring the relationship between thumb-sucking and psychopathology. J Pediatr Psychol 19:431–441, 1994

Friman PC, Handwerk ML, Swearer SM, et al: Do children with primary nocturnal enuresis have clinically significant behavior problems? Arch Pediatr Adolesc Med 152:537–539, 1998

Friman PC, Byrd MR, Oksol EM: Characteristics of oral-digital habits, in Tic Disorders, Trichotillomania, and Other Repetitive Behavior Disorders: Behavioral Approaches to Analysis and Treatment. Edited by Woods DW, Miltenberger RG. New York, Springer, 2006, pp 197–222

Goldman S, Wang C, Salgado MW, et al: Motor stereotypies in children with autism and other developmental disorders. Child Neurol 51:30–38, 2008

Hadley NH: Fingernail Biting. New York, Spectrum, 1984

Hall S, Oliver C, Murphy G: Early development of self-injurious behavior: an empirical study. Am J Ment Retard 106:189–199, 2001

Hall S, Thorns T, Oliver C: Structural and environmental characteristics of stereotyped behaviors. Am J Ment Retard 108:391–402, 2003

Hansen DJ, Tishelman AC, Hawkins RP, et al: Habits with potential as disorders: prevalence, severity, and other characteristics among college students. Behav Modif 14:66–80, 1990

Hashizume Y, Yoshijima H, Uchimura N, et al: Case of head banging that continued to adolescence. Psychiatry Clin Neurosci 56:255–256, 2002

Infante PF: An epidemiological study of finger habits in preschool children, as related to malocclusion, socioeconomic status, race, sex, and size of community. J Dent Child 43:33–38, 1976

Iorizzo M, Piraccini BM, Tosti A: Nail cosmetics in nail disorders. J Cosmet Dermatol 6:53–58, 2007

Iwata BA, Dorsey MF, Slifer KJ, et al: Toward a functional analysis of self-injury. J Appl Behav Anal 27:197–209, 1994

Jackson MA, Hughes RC, Ward SP, et al: "Headbanging" and carotid dissection. Br Med J (Clin Res Ed) 287:1262, 1983

Joubert CE: Relationship of self-esteem, manifest anxiety, and obsessive-compulsiveness to personal habits. Psychol Rep 73:579–583, 1993

Klackenberg B: Thumb sucking: frequency and etiology. Pediatrics 4:418–424, 1949

Kravitz H, Boehm JJ: Rhythmic habit patterns in infancy. Child Dev 42:399–413, 1971

Leekam S, Tandos J, McConachie H, et al: Repetitive behaviors in typically developing 2-year-olds. J Child Psychol Psychiatry 48:1131–1138, 2007

Leung KC, Robson WL: Nail biting. Clin Pediatr 29:690–692, 1990

MacLean WE Jr, Ellis DN, Galbreath HN, et al: Rhythmic motor behavior of preambulatory motor impaired, Down syndrome and nondisabled children: a comparative analysis. J Abnorm Child Psychol 19:319–330, 1991

Mahalski PA: The incidence of attachment objects and oral habits at bedtime in two longitudinal samples of children aged 1.5–7 years. J Child Psychol Psychiatry 24:283–295, 1983

Mahalski PA, Stanton WR: The relationship between digit sucking and behavior problems: a longitudinal study over 10 years. J Child Psychol Psychiatry 33:913–923, 1992

Mahone EM, Bridges D, Prahme C, et al: Repetitive arm and hand movements (complex motor stereotypies) in children. J Pediatr 145:391–395, 2004

Malone AJ, Massler M: Index of nailbiting in children. J Abnorm Soc Psychol 47:193–202, 1952

Massler M, Malone AJ: Nail-biting: a review. J Pediatr 36:523, 1950

Medoff-Cooper B, Shults J, Kaplan J: Sucking behavior of preterm neonates as a predictor of developmental outcomes. J Dev Behav Pediatr 30:16–22, 2009

Moore GJ, McNeill RW, D'Anna JA: The effects of digit sucking on facial growth. J Am Dent Assoc 84:592–599, 1972

Muthugovindan D, Singer H: Motor stereotypy disorders. Curr Opin Neurol 22:131–136, 2009

Nijhof G, Joha D, Pekelharing H: Aspects of stereotypic behaviour among autistic persons: a study of the literature. The British Journal of Developmental Disabilities 44:3–13, 1998

Odenrick L, Brattstrom V: Nail biting: frequency and association with root resorption during orthodontic treatment. Br J Orthod 12:78–81, 1985

Ozturk M, Ozturk OM: Thumb sucking and falling asleep. Br J Med Psychol 50:95–103, 1977

Pennington LA: Incidence of nail biting among adults. Am J Psychiatry 102:241–245, 1945

Peterson JE: Pediatric oral habits, in Pediatric Dentistry: Scientific Foundations and Clinical Practice. Edited by Stewart RE, Barber TK, Troutman KD, et al. St Louis, MO, CV Mosby, 1982, pp 361–372

Popovich F, Thompson GW: Thumb and finger sucking: analysis of contributory factors in 1258 children. Can J Public Health 65:277–280, 1974

Rankin EA, Jabaley ME, Blair SJ, et al: Acquired rotational digital deformity in children as a result of finger sucking. J Hand Surg 13:535–539, 1988

Richler J, Bishop SL, Kleinke JR, et al: Restricted and repetitive behaviors in young children with autism spectrum disorders. J Autism Dev Disord 37:73–85, 2007

Robey KL, Reck JF, Giacomini KD, et al: Modes and patterns of self-mutilation in persons with Lesch-Nyhan disease. Dev Med Child Neurol 45:167–171, 2003

Sallustro F, Atwell CW: Body rocking, head banging, and head rolling in normal children. Pediatrics 93:704–708, 1978

Samman PD: Nail disorders caused by external influences. J Soc Cosmet Chem 28:351–353, 1977

Schwartz SS, Gallagher RJ, Berkson G: Normal repetitive and abnormal stereotyped behavior of nonretarded infants and young mentally retarded children. Am J Ment Defic 90:625–630, 1986

Silber KP, Haynes CE: Treating nail biting: a comparative analysis of mild aversion and competing response therapies. Behav Res Ther 30:15–22, 1992

Spalter HF, Bemporad JR, Sours JA: Cataracts following chronic headbanging. Arch Ophthalmol 83:182–186, 1970

Symons FJ, Clark RD, Hatton DD, et al: Self-injurious behavior in young boys with fragile X syndrome. Am J Med Genet A 118:115–121, 2003

Thelen E: Rhythmical stereotypies in normal human infants. Anim Behav 27:699–715, 1979

Thelen E: Rhythmical behavior in infancy: an ethological perspective. Dev Psychol 17:237–257, 1981

Thelen E: Normal infant stereotypies: a dynamic systems approach, in Stereotypies: Brain-Behavior Relationships. Edited by Sprague RL, Newell KM. Washington, DC, American Psychological Association, 1996, pp 139–165

Troster H: Prevalence and functions of stereotyped behaviors in nonhandicapped children in residential care. J Abnorm Child Psychol 22:79–97, 1994

Turbeville DF, Fearnow RG: Is it possible to identify the child who is a "high risk" candidate for the accidental ingestion of a poison? Clin Pediatr (Phila) 15:918–919, 1976

Vogel LD: When children put their fingers in their mouths: should parents and dentists care? N Y State Dent J 64:48–53, 1998

Walker BA, Ziskind E: Relationship of nail biting to sociopathy. J Nerv Ment Dis 164:64–65, 1977

Warren JJ, Bishara SE, Steinbock KL, et al: Effects of oral habits' duration on dental characteristics in the primary dentition. J Am Dent Assoc 132:1685–1693, 2001

Wechsler D: The incidence and significance of fingernail biting in children. Psychoanal Rev 18:201–209, 1931

Wehmeyer ML: Typical and atypical repetitive motor behaviors in young children at risk for severe mental retardation. Am J Ment Retard 96:53–62, 1991

Wehmeyer ML: Factors related to the expression of typical and atypical repetitive movements of young children with mental retardation. International Journal of Disability, Development, and Education 41:33–49, 1994

Weinlander MM, Lee SH: Suicidal age and childhood onychophagia among neurotic veterans. J Clin Psychol 34:31–32, 1978

Wells JH, Haines J, Williams CL: Severe morbid onychophagia: the classification as self-mutilation and a proposed model of maintenance. Aust N Z J Psychiatry 32:534–545, 1998

Werry JS, Carlielle J, Fitzpatrick J: Rhythmic motor activities (stereotypies) in children under five: etiology and prevalence. J Am Acad Child Psychiatry 22:329–336, 1983

Woods DW, Miltenberger RG: Are persons with nervous habits nervous? A preliminary examination of habit function in a nonreferred population. J Appl Behav Anal 29:259–261, 1996

Woods DW, Miltenberger RG, Flach AD: Habits, tics, and stuttering: prevalence and relation to anxiety and somatic awareness. Behav Modif 20:216–225, 1996

PSYCHOBIOLOGY OF HAIR-PULLING DISORDER (TRICHOTILLOMANIA) AND SKIN-PICKING DISORDER

Dan J. Stein, M.D., Ph.D.
Christine Lochner, Ph.D.

Hair pulling, skin picking, and other body-focused stereotypic disorders are, on the one hand, simply motoric actions. Thus the psychobiology of these behaviors might overlap with that of any motoric action and not be deserving of study in its own right. Hair-pulling disorder (trichotillomania), skin-picking disorder, and other body-focused stereotypic disorders, on the other hand, constitute psychiatric syndromes with constellations of affective, conative, cognitive, and motoric symptoms. It would not be surprising, for example, if such conditions represent "grooming disorders," or disruptions of behavioral sequences that are present in a range of species and have an evolved function (Feusner et al. 2009; Stein et al. 1994a). Investigation of the psychobiology of such conditions not only may be relevant to optimizing their treatment but also may shed light on a range of psychiatric disorders with overlapping affective, conative, cognitive, or motoric symptoms.

In this chapter, we summarize research on the psychobiology of trichotillomania and skin-picking disorder and argue that although significant advances have been made, additional work is needed in order to fulfill the potential the psychobiology of trichotillomania and skin-picking disorder may have for illuminating a range of other disorders.

COGNITIVE-AFFECTIVE PROCESSES

A cognitive-affective neuroscience approach to psychiatric disorders may usefully begin by considering whether any particular cognitive-affective processes characteristically mediate the disorder (Stein et al. 2000, 2006). Current work on delineating endophenotypes relevant to psychiatric disorders also potentially provides various leads for considering processes that may be relevant to a condition such as trichotillomania (Gottesman and Gould 2003). In this section, we outline a number of possibly relevant cognitive-affective processes. In subsequent sections, we discuss the neural circuits involved in these processes and the molecular systems that may be particularly relevant in that neurocircuitry.

A first set of processes that may be relevant to trichotillomania and other body-focused repetitive behaviors (BFRBs) comprises those involved in responding to stressors and other negative stimuli. Clinical research has found relatively high rates of early adversity in subjects with trichotillomania (Christenson et al. 1991; Lochner et al. 2002) as well as in subjects with a range of stereotypic self-injurious behaviors (Schroeder et al. 2001). There are also data that hair pulling is triggered by a range of negative affects, ranging from those that are experienced as more arousing (e.g., anxiety) to those experienced as entailing insufficient levels of arousal (e.g., boredom) (Christenson et al. 1993). Similar triggers are present in skin picking and other stereotypic disorders (Bohne et al. 2005a). In response to such negative affects, stereotypic behaviors can release tension or lead to a sense of relief, rather than pain, at least in the short term. Over the longer term, however, psychosocial impairment due to such behaviors may contribute to the burden of stressors.

A second set of processes that may be relevant to trichotillomania and other BFRBs constitutes those involved in reward-driven repetitive behaviors. Hair pulling is often reported as pleasurable, and it is notable that in patients with obsessive-compulsive disorder (OCD), comorbid trichotillomania clusters together with conditions such as pathological gambling and hypersexual disorder (Lochner et al. 2005). Alterations in reward processes may be relevant to understanding a wide range of repetitive behaviors, including both simple motoric acts and more complex stereotypic behaviors, as well as diverse psychiatric conditions, ranging from more impulsive conditions (e.g., substance use, pathological gambling, and other presumptive behavioral addictions) to compulsive conditions (e.g., obsessive-compulsive and spectrum disorders) (Fineberg et al. 2010).

A third set of processes that may be relevant to trichotillomania and other BFRBs comprises those involved in disrupted control of behavior. Again, there is growing understanding of the nature of control mechanisms, ranging from those involved in control of simple motoric actions to those involved in more complex decision making. In psychiatry, disruption of simple motoric actions is seen in conditions such as Tourette syndrome, whereas symptoms indicative of executive dyscontrol are seen in a broad range of illnesses, again including both impulsive and compulsive disorders. Such observations have contributed to the notion of a compulsive-impulsive spectrum of disorders characterized by unwanted repetitive behaviors (Stein 2000), although current thinking suggests that multiple orthogonal dimensions may be required to map relationships between such conditions (Stein and Lochner 2006).

NEURAL CIRCUITRY

Basic Science

A range of neural circuitry is involved in responding to stressors and in maintaining optimal levels of arousal. In particular, there is growing information about the role of limbic structures in mediating negative affects. For example, basic laboratory work has demonstrated that after processing by sensory pathways (moving from peripheral neurons to central relay stations such as the thalamus), the amygdala plays a key coordinating role, sending efferent fibers to a range of regions involved in the fight-or-flight response, including the hypothalamus and brain stem (Le Doux 1998).

Various neuronal circuits are involved in mediating seemingly driven repetitive behaviors. In particular, there is evidence that the neural circuitry involved in reward processing plays a role here. For example, basic research has demonstrated that the nucleus accumbens plays a key role in processing reward, and clinical research has indicated that the ventral striatum is implicated in a range of unwanted repetitive behaviors seen in psychiatric disorders, including pathological gambling and substance use disorders (Chambers et al. 2003; Grant et al. 2006).

Prefrontal cortex and descending neurons to a range of subcortical structures play a key role in executive control. In particular, frontal-striatal circuits seem to be involved in a range of control mechanisms. For example, frontal-striatal circuitry is disrupted in both impulsive disorders (where there may be decreased prefrontal control) and compulsive conditions (where there may be compensatory increases in activity in frontostriatal circuitry) (Stein 2000). The cerebellum also plays a key role in a number of control processes, both motoric and cognitive (Berntson et al. 1973).

The animal literature on the neuroanatomy of grooming and other stereotypic behaviors points to the involvement of some of these same neural circuits (Cooper and Dourish 1990; Ridley 1994). In particular, the striatum plays a key role in governing innate motor programs (MacLean 1973). Early adversity is associated with altered striatal cytoarchitecture and thus perhaps with increased release of such programs (Martin et al. 1991). It is also notable that chronic stress leads to opposing structural changes in the associative and sensorimotor corticostriatal circuits underlying different behavioral strategies, with atrophy of medial prefrontal cortex and the associative striatum but hypertrophy of the sensorimotor striatum, so that after stress, strategies become biased toward the habitual (Dias-Ferreira et al. 2009).

Neuropsychology

The clinical literature provides few cases in which neural lesions have led to trichotillomania or other BFRBs (McGrath et al. 2002). Early suggestions that some trichotillomania patients may overlap with patients with pediatric autoimmune neuropsychiatric disorders associated with streptococcal infections in having anti-striatal antibodies after streptococcal infection (Stein et al. 1997b) have not been supported. There is also little evidence of increased neurological soft signs in patients with trichotillomania (Stein et al. 1994b). There is, however, a growing body of work documenting specific impairment in neuropsychological tasks in this disorder, recently reviewed carefully by Chamberlain et al. (2009), and we turn to this next.

Early work employed batteries of neuropsychological tasks to study trichotillomania (Bohne et al. 2005b; Coetzer and Stein 1999; Keuthen et al. 1996; Martin et al. 1993; Rettew et al. 1991; Stanley et al. 1997). Taken together, this early work found inconsistent evidence of executive and visual-spatial dysfunctions—that is, a number of studies showed deficits in these domains in patients with trichotillomania compared with healthy control subjects, but there was also little consistency across studies, with different tasks employed or different findings when the same task was studied. This early work also pointed to differences in the profile of neuropsychological impairments between trichotillomania and OCD.

More recent work has focused on specific tasks thought relevant to elucidating key cognitive-affective processes or endophenotypes thought relevant to trichotillomania (Bohne et al. 2008; Chamberlain et al. 2006a, 2006b, 2007). For example, a stop-signal task thought to reflect motor inhibitory control was found to be more impaired in individuals with trichotillomania than in healthy control subjects, with OCD subjects demonstrating intermediate values (Chamberlain et al. 2006b). In contrast, trichotillomania patients did not differ from healthy control subjects on a task assessing cognitive flexibility, whereas OCD patients were significantly impaired (Chamberlain et al. 2006b). It is notable that patients with skin-picking disorder show a similar pattern to those with trichotillomania on these tasks (Odlaug et al. 2010).

Nevertheless, the relationship between such putative neuropsychological abnormalities in trichotillomania and hair-pulling symptoms and comorbid psychopathology remains unclear, and similarly it is uncertain whether these neuropsychological abnormalities are present in those at risk for developing trichotillomania (e.g., first-degree relatives). Small-animal studies have documented neuropsychological deficits in models relevant to trichotillomania; for example, Garner and Mason (2002) found that vole stereotypies correlated with inappropriate responding in extinction learning, impairments of response timing, and other evidence of striatal disinhibition of response selection; further research in this area may also be productive. Ultimately, neuropsychological impairments may be a useful target for treatment development (Chamberlain et al. 2010a).

Brain Imaging

A number of structural and functional brain imaging studies of trichotillomania are now available. Early work suggested that trichotillomania might be associated with decreased striatal volume, particularly of the left putamen (O'Sullivan et al. 1997), as well as reduced left inferior frontal cortex volume (Grachev 1997). However, other work either did not find striatal differences between patients with trichotillomania and healthy control subjects (Stein et al. 1997a) or pointed to reduced volume of other regions such as the cerebellum (Keuthen et al. 2007).

A recent study using voxel-based morphometry concluded that patients with trichotillomania had increased gray matter density in the left caudate-putamen and left amygdala-hippocampal formation, bilateral cingulate, and right frontal cortices—regions that the authors pointed out are involved in affect regulation, motor habits, and top-down cognition (Chamberlain et al. 2008). A diffusion tensor imaging study also indicated altered white matter in trichotillomania, with significantly reduced fractional anisotropy in the anterior cingulate, pre-supplementary motor area, and temporal cortices (Chamberlain et al. 2010b).

Functional work with positron emission tomography (PET) and single-photon emission computed tomography (SPECT) has similarly suggested localized abnormalities in cerebral metabolism and perfusion in trichotillomania. Regions that have been implicated in such work include the cerebellum and parietal cortex (Swedo et al. 1991) and the temporal cortex (Vythilingum et al. 2002). A functional magnetic resonance imaging study found no evidence of abnormal brain activation during implicit learning in trichotillomania, consistent with normal striatal function (Rauch et al. 2007). However, treatment of trichotillomania with a selective serotonin reuptake inhibitor (SSRI) led to reduced activity in frontal cortical regions, the left putamen, and the right anterior temporal lobe on SPECT (Stein et al. 2002), partially consistent with structural findings that have emphasized the role of frontostriatal circuitry in this condition.

This body of work on trichotillomania, however, comprises only a few studies, each with relatively few subjects, and with little independent replication of findings. Given advances in magnetic resonance spectroscopy, diffusion tensor imaging, and molecular imaging, it is hopefully only a matter of time before such methodologies are more widely applied to hair pulling and other BFRBs. It would be useful to use functional magnetic resonance imaging to assess stress response and affect regulation, habit and reward processing, and executive dyscontrol in trichotillomania. In the interim, however, it is possible to conclude that there is limited evidence from brain imaging for the involvement of various brain regions, consistent with cognitive-affective processes hypothesized to be involved in hair pulling, particularly those involved in affect regulation, habit formation, and executive control.

MOLECULAR NEUROSCIENCE

Neurotransmitter and Neuropeptide Systems

Several different molecular systems are thought to be relevant to the cognitive-affective processes and neuronal circuitry that may be involved in trichotillomania and other BFRBs. Here we review work on monoaminergic systems (e.g., the serotonin, dopamine, and norepinephrine systems), on amino acid neurotransmitter systems (e.g., the glutamate system), and on neuropeptide systems (e.g., the opioid system). Although there is insufficient space here to cover the neurobiology of the stereotypic self-injurious behaviors seen in a broad range of developmental disorders (e.g., Prader-Willi syndrome, Lesch-Nyhan syndrome, Cornelia de Lange syndrome), it is worth noting that study of such conditions may also shed light on pathways relevant to hair-pulling and skin-picking disorders (Stein and Simeon 1998).

An early study of 5-hydroxyindoleacetic acid in the cerebrospinal fluid of trichotillomania patients suggested that this was normal but nevertheless predicted response to pharmacotherapy with a serotonin reuptake inhibitor (Ninan et al. 1992). Pharmacological challenge of trichotillomania patients with a serotonin agonist provided some evidence of an abnormal behavioral response compared with control subjects, although there were no differences in neuroendocrine response (Stein et al. 1995). Selective response to serotonin reuptake inhibitors provided an indirect signal of serotonergic involvement, and another early study provided significant impetus to the field by indicating that trichotillomania and nail biting, and possibly stereotypic movement disorder and self-injurious stereotypies, may respond more robustly to clomipramine than desipramine (Castellanos et al. 1996; Leonard et al. 1991; Lewis et al. 1996; Swedo 1989). This is also consistent with basic work on the role of serotonin in grooming and repetitive behavior (Cooper and Dourish 1990) as well as the pharmacotherapeutic response of animal stereotypies (Hugo et al. 2003; Korff et al. 2008) and pathological grooming (Rapoport et al. 1992; Seibert et al. 2004; Stein et al. 1998) to serotonin reuptake inhibitors. Nevertheless, subsequent work on response of trichotillomania and skin-picking disorder to these medications has been relatively disappointing (see Chapter 12, "Pharmacotherapy").

There is relatively little direct evidence of the involvement of the dopamine system in trichotillomania and other BFRBs. Nevertheless, a large body of animal work points to the role of the dopamine system in stereotypic and grooming behaviors (Berridge et al. 2005; Cooper and Dourish 1990; Iglauer and Rasim 1993; Korff et al. 2008). Furthermore, stereotypic symptoms, including hair pulling and skin picking, may be seen clinically after administration of psychostimulants that increase dopaminergic activity (Martin et al. 1998). Conversely, there is evidence that hair pulling, skin picking, and a range of stereotypic self-injurious behaviors respond to treatment with dopamine blockers (Stein and Hollander 1992; Stein et al. 1998; Van Ameringen et al. 1999, 2006).

The norepinephrine system has not been well studied in trichotillomania and other BFRBs. However, it has been suggested that abnormalities in the stop-signal response in trichotillomania may reflect involvement of the norepinephrine system in trichotillomania (Chamberlain et al. 2009). Modafinil, which promotes low-tonic/high-phasic locus coeruleus–noradrenergic activity, did not, however, improve motor inhibitory control or other cognitive functions in trichotillomania in a single-dose paradigm (Chamberlain et al. 2010a).

There is limited work on the involvement of the glutamate or γ-aminobutyric acid (GABA) systems in trichotillomania and other BFRBs. Nevertheless, there are anecdotal reports of hair pulling responding to *N*-acetylcysteine, and a placebo-controlled trial in trichotillomania yielded exciting positive data for this amino acid (Grant et al. 2009). *N*-Acetylcysteine administration leads to cystine uptake, which in turn leads to the reverse transport of glutamate into the extracellular space, thus stimulating inhibitory metabotropic glutamate receptors and reducing synaptic release of glutamate. The authors suggested that *N*-acetylcysteine may target prefrontal glutamatergic efferents to the nucleus accumbens, thus decreasing repetitive behaviors. In addition, however, they noted that it may be protective to glial cell functioning during hyperglutamatergic states and may usefully enhance glial uptake of glutamate by excitatory amino acid transporters (Grant et al. 2009). It is also notable that lamotrigine, which also acts on the glutamate system, may be helpful in a subset of skin-picking patients with relatively impaired cognitive flexibility (Grant et al. 2010).

There is a body of work suggesting that the opioid system is involved in self-injurious behaviors (Herman 1990; Symons et al. 2004). Furthermore, there is a literature implicating opioid systems in animal grooming and stereotypies (Dodman et al. 1997; Schroeder et al. 2008). There is, however, little evidence of altered pain processing in patients with trichotillomania (Christenson et al. 1994). Early open-label research suggested that trichotillomania may respond to naltrexone (O'Sullivan et al. 1999). However, this body of work is relatively sparse, and no studies have used PET radioligands to directly examine opioid receptors in patients with this disorder. Similarly, although it might be hypothesized that corticotropin-releasing factor or oxytocin is implicated in stress responses in trichotillomania and other BFRBs (Leckman et al. 1994); that gonadal hormones may be relevant to understanding why trichotillomania is more common in females, typically begins at menarche, and is exacerbated premenstrually (Keuthen et al. 1997); or that cutaneous neuropeptides play a role in BFRBs (O'Sullivan et al. 1998), there are few empirical data to shed light on these issues.

Family and Genetic Studies

Family and genetic studies provide the potential of exploring a broader range of molecular systems that may be involved in trichotillomania and other BFRBs. Data indicating heritability of trichotillomania would allow exploration of particular inherited variants in patients with this disorder. Alternatively, studies of gene-environment interactions in these patients might allow exploration of the way in which particular variants and particular environments interact to result in hair-pulling behaviors.

There is high comorbidity of different BFRBs and some evidence that such disorders are more likely seen in OCD than in other psychiatric disorders (Lochner and Stein 2010; Richter et al. 2003). Although relatively few studies have explored the prevalence of hair pulling or skin picking in family members of probands with trichotillomania, skin-picking disorder, or OCD (Bienvenu et al. 2000; Christenson et al. 1992; Lenane et al. 1992), such work has provided support for grooming disorders as part of the familial OCD spectrum. Furthermore, a twin study has found that monozygotic twins have higher concordance of trichotillomania than do dizygotic twins (Novak et al. 2009). Thus, although heritability is likely only modest, such work does encourage further studies of the genetic bases of trichotillomania and other BFRBs.

Such genetic work has, however, been limited to only a few studies, all of which have employed gene association methods. This work has suggested involvement of variants in particular serotonergic genes (Hemmings et al. 2006), *SLITRK1* (SLIT and NTRK-like family, member 1) (Zuchner et al. 2006), and *SAPAP3* (synapse-associated protein 90 [SAP90]/postsynaptic density-95 [PSD95]–associated protein 3) (Zuchner et al. 2009). Nevertheless, sample sizes are small, and there have been insufficient replications to make this work anything more than preliminary (Boardman et al. 2011). It is notable, however, that work on *SAPAP3* variants in trichotillomania derived from earlier laboratory work; mice deficient in postsynaptic *SAPAP3* develop a phenotype that includes compulsive grooming and increased anxiety and are rescued by the administration of SSRIs (Welch et al. 2007).

From Bench to Bedside

Indeed, animal work may ultimately play a key role in informing our understanding of the psychobiology of trichotillomania. A long tradition of animal work on the neuroscience of habits and stereotypies is clearly relevant to understanding trichotillomania and other BFRBs (Berridge et al. 2005; Korff et al. 2008). Grooming behaviors, including hair pulling itself (Reinhardt 2005), barbering (Garner et al. 2004; Kalueff et al. 2006), and feather picking (Bordnick et al. 1994; Garner et al. 2003; Grindlinger and Ramsay 1991; Jenkins 2001; Seibert et al. 2004), seem to have particular face validity for trichotillomania. There have been a number of particularly interesting developments in this area in recent years.

Thus, for example, Greer and Capecchi (2002) reported that mice with mutations in *Hoxb8* demonstrated excessive grooming with hair removal and skin lesions and that *Hoxb8* is expressed in brain regions implicated in animal grooming and in human OCD (orbital cortex, anterior cingulate, striatum, and limbic system). More recently, they found these animals had abnormal microglia and that such microglia derived from bone marrow cells, so that transplantation of wild-type bone marrow into *Hoxb8* mutant mice restored normal function (Chen et al. 2010). This work provides novel insights into the close relationship between the immune and central nervous systems, which may ultimately be relevant to understanding a broad range of disorders.

More generally, animal work may be useful in understanding how stressors exacerbate habits (Dias-Ferreira et al. 2009), how behavioral addictions emerge (Fineberg et al. 2010), and how behavioral dyscontrol occurs (Dalley et al. 2004). At the same time, however, there have been important difficulties in moving from bench to bedside. In particular, although the possibility remains open that animal models are able to shed light on particular cognitive-affective processes, neural circuitry, or molecular mechanisms in hair pulling and other BFRBs, there is ultimately a significant gap between what is seen at the bench and the complexity of human psychopathology. Such complexity reflects in part the subjective complexity of human experience (consider, for example, the distinction between automatic and focused hair pulling) as well as the potential complexity of human psychobiological mechanisms (given important differences in neuronal and molecular structures between *Homo sapiens* and laboratory species).

CONCLUSION

On the one hand, the psychobiology of trichotillomania and other BFRBs has received growing interest in recent years, with studies employing increasing methodological sophistication and work ranging from animal models to genetic and brain imaging studies. A number of possible cognitive-affective processes relevant to these conditions have been identified, and the relevant neural circuitry and molecular systems have been delineated. Furthermore, important links have been made between the bench and bedside in the attempt to understand these conditions. This represents enormous progress, with implications not only for hair pulling and skin picking but also for obsessive-compulsive spectrum disorders and, on occasion, for a range of other psychiatric conditions.

On the other hand, there is a relative paucity of data on the psychobiology of trichotillomania and other BFRBs. The total number of studies on the cognitive-affective neuroscience of these conditions is relatively small, and the total number of subjects studied to date is also quite modest. Thus key issues, such as establishing links between psychobiological mechanisms, trichotillomania and skin-picking subtypes, and treatment outcomes, have not been possible to explore. Furthermore, available methodologies (e.g., gene arrays, PET radioligands) and designs (e.g., gene-environment interactions, imaging after psychotherapy) have not yet been applied to these conditions. Much additional work is needed on both the distal (evolutionary) and proximal (psychobiological) mechanisms underlying grooming and stereotypic behaviors and symptoms. Such work will hopefully emerge over the next decades.

REFERENCES

Berntson GG, Potolicchio SJ Jr, Miller NE: Evidence for higher functions of the cerebellum: eating and grooming elicited by cerebellar stimulation in cats. Proc Natl Acad Sci USA 70:2497–2499, 1973

Berridge KC, Aldridge JW, Houchard KR, et al: Sequential super-stereotypy of an instinctive fixed action pattern in hyper-dopaminergic mutant mice: a model of obsessive compulsive disorder and Tourette's. BMC Biol 3:4, 2005

Bienvenu OJ, Samuels JF, Riddle MA, et al: The relationship of obsessive-compulsive disorder to possible spectrum disorders: results from a family study. Biol Psychiatry 48:287–293, 2000

Boardman L, van der Merwe L, Lochner C, et al: Investigating SAPAP3 variants in the etiology of obsessive-compulsive disorder and trichotillomania in the South African white population. Compr Psychiatry 52:181–187, 2011

Bohne A, Keuthen N, Wilhelm S: Pathologic hairpulling, skin picking, and nail biting. Ann Clin Psychiatry 17:227–232, 2005a

Bohne A, Savage CR, Deckersbach T, et al: Visuospatial abilities, memory, and executive functioning in trichotillomania and obsessive-compulsive disorder. J Clin Exp Neuropsychol 27:385–399, 2005b

Bohne A, Savage CR, Deckersbach T, et al: Motor inhibition in trichotillomania and obsessive-compulsive disorder. J Psychiatr Res 42:141–150, 2008

Bordnick PS, Thyer BA, Ritchie BW: Feather picking disorder and trichotillomania: an avian model of human psychopathology. J Behav Ther Exp Psychiatry 25:189–196, 1994

Castellanos FX, Ritchie GF, Marsh WL, et al: DSM-IV stereotypic movement disorder: persistence of stereotypies of infancy in intellectually normal adolescents and adults. J Clin Psychiatry 57:116–122, 1996

Chamberlain SR, Blackwell AD, Fineberg NA, et al: Strategy implementation in obsessive-compulsive disorder and trichotillomania. Psychol Med 36:91–97, 2006a

Chamberlain SR, Fineberg NA, Blackwell AD, et al: Motor inhibition and cognitive flexibility in obsessive-compulsive disorder and trichotillomania. Am J Psychiatry 163:1282–1284, 2006b

Chamberlain SR, Fineberg NA, Blackwell AD, et al: A neuropsychological comparison of obsessive-compulsive disorder and trichotillomania. Neuropsychologia 45:654–662, 2007

Chamberlain SR, Menzies LA, Fineberg NA, et al: Grey matter abnormalities in trichotillomania: morphometric magnetic resonance imaging study. Br J Psychiatry 193:216–221, 2008

Chamberlain SR, Odlaug BL, Boulougouris V, et al: Trichotillomania: neurobiology and treatment. Neurosci Biobehav Rev 33:831–842, 2009

Chamberlain SR, Grant JE, Costa A, et al: Effects of acute modafinil on cognition in trichotillomania. Psychopharmacology (Berl) 212:597–601, 2010a

Chamberlain SR, Hampshire A, Menzies LA, et al: Reduced brain white matter integrity in trichotillomania: a diffusion tensor imaging study. Arch Gen Psychiatry 67:965–971, 2010b

Chambers RA, Taylor JR, Potenza MN: Developmental neurocircuitry of motivation in adolescence: a critical period of addiction vulnerability. Am J Psychiatry 160:1041–1052, 2003

Chen SK, Tvrdik P, Peden E, et al: Hematopoietic origin of pathological grooming in Hoxb8 mutant mice. Cell 141:775–785, 2010

Christenson GA, Mackenzie TB, Mitchell JE: Characteristics of 60 adult chronic hair pullers. Am J Psychiatry 148:365–370, 1991

Christenson GA, Mackenzie TB, Reeve EA: Familial trichotillomania (letter). Am J Psychiatry 149:283, 1992

Christenson GA, Ristvedt SL, Mackenzie TB: Identification of trichotillomania cue profiles. Behav Res Ther 31:315–320, 1993

Christenson GA, Raymond NC, Faris PL, et al: Pain thresholds are not elevated in trichotillomania. Biol Psychiatry 36:347–349, 1994

Coetzer R, Stein DJ: Neuropsychological measures in women with obsessive-compulsive disorder and trichotillomania. Psychiatry Clin Neurosci 53:413–415, 1999

Cooper SJ, Dourish CT: Neurobiology of Stereotyped Behaviour. Oxford, UK, Clarendon Press/Oxford University Press, 1990

Dalley JW, Cardinal RN, Robbins TW: Prefrontal executive and cognitive functions in rodents: neural and neurochemical substrates. Neurosci Biobehav Rev 28:771–784, 2004

Dias-Ferreira E, Sousa JC, Melo I, et al: Chronic stress causes frontostriatal reorganization and affects decision-making. Science 325:621–625, 2009

Dodman NH, Moon-Fanelli A, Mertens PA, et al: Animal models of obsessive-compulsive disorder, in Obsessive-Compulsive Disorders: Diagnosis, Etiology, Treatment. Edited by Hollander E, Stein DJ. New York, Marcel Dekker, 1997

Feusner JD, Hembacher E, Phillips KA: The mouse who couldn't stop washing: pathologic grooming in animals and humans. CNS Spectr 14:503–513, 2009

Fineberg NA, Potenza MN, Chamberlain SR, et al: Probing compulsive and impulsive behaviors, from animal models to endophenotypes: a narrative review. Neuropsychopharmacology 35:591–604, 2010

Garner JP, Mason GJ: Evidence for a relationship between cage stereotypies and behavioural disinhibition in laboratory rodents. Behav Brain Res 136:83–92, 2002

Garner JP, Meehan CL, Mench JA: Stereotypies in caged parrots, schizophrenia and autism: evidence for a common mechanism. Behav Brain Res 145:125–134, 2003

Garner JP, Weisker SM, Dufour B, et al: Barbering (fur and whisker trimming) by laboratory mice as a model of human trichotillomania and obsessive-compulsive spectrum disorders. Comp Med 54:216–224, 2004

Gottesman II, Gould TD: The endophenotype concept in psychiatry: etymology and strategic intentions. Am J Psychiatry 160:636–645, 2003

Grachev ID: MRI-based morphometric topographic parcellation of human neocortex in trichotillomania. Psychiatry Clin Neurosci 51:315–321, 1997

Grant JE, Brewer JA, Potenza MN: The neurobiology of substance and behavioral addictions. CNS Spectr 11:924–930, 2006

Grant JE, Odlaug BL, Kim SW: N-Acetylcysteine, a glutamate modulator, in the treatment of trichotillomania a double-blind, placebo-controlled study. Arch Gen Psychiatry 66:756–763, 2009

Grant JE, Odlaug BL, Chamberlain SR, et al: A double-blind, placebo-controlled trial of lamotrigine for pathological skin picking: treatment efficacy and neurocognitive predictors of response. J Clin Psychopharmacol 30:396–403, 2010

Greer JM, Capecchi MR: Hoxb8 is required for normal grooming behavior in mice. Neuron 33:23–34, 2002

Grindlinger HM, Ramsay E: Compulsive feather picking in birds. Arch Gen Psychiatry 48:857, 1991

Hemmings SMJ, Kinnear CJ, Lochner C, et al: Genetic correlates in trichotillomania: a case-control association study in the South African Caucasian population. Isr J Psychiatry Relat Sci 43:93–101, 2006

Herman BH: A possible role of proopiomelanocortin peptides in self-injurious behavior. Prog Neuropsychopharmacol Biol Psychiatry 14(suppl):S109–S139, 1990

Hugo C, Seier J, Mdhluli C, et al: Fluoxetine decreases stereotypic behavior in primates. Prog Neuropsychopharmacol Biol Psychiatry 27:639–643, 2003

Iglauer F, Rasim R: Treatment of psychogenic feather picking in psittacine birds with a dopamine antagonist. J Small Anim Pract 34:564–566, 1993

Jenkins JR: Feather picking and self-mutilation in psittacine birds. Vet Clin North Am Exot Anim Pract 4:651–667, 2001

Kalueff AV, Minasyan A, Keisala T, et al: Hair barbering in mice: implications for neurobehavioural research. Behav Processes 71:8–15, 2006

Keuthen NJ, Savage CR, O'Sullivan RL, et al: Neuropsychological functioning in trichotillomania. Biol Psychiatry 39:747–749, 1996

Keuthen NJ, O'Sullivan RL, Hayday CF, et al: The relationship of menstrual cycle and pregnancy to compulsive hairpulling. Psychother Psychosom 66:33–37, 1997

Keuthen NJ, Makris N, Schlerf JE, et al: Evidence for reduced cerebellar volumes in trichotillomania. Biol Psychiatry 61:374–381, 2007

Korff S, Stein DJ, Harvey BH: Stereotypic behaviour in the deer mouse: pharmacological validation and relevance for obsessive compulsive disorder. Prog Neuropsychopharmacol Biol Psychiatry 32:348–355, 2008

Leckman JF, Goodman WK, North WG: The role of central oxytocin in obsessive compulsive disorder and related normal behavior. Psychoneuroendocrinology 19:723–749, 1994

Le Doux J: Fear and the brain: where have we been, and where are we going? Biol Psychiatry 44:1229–1238, 1998

Lenane MC, Swedo SE, Rapoport JL, et al: Rates of obsessive-compulsive disorder in 1st degree relatives of patients with trichotillomania: a research note. J Child Psychol Psychiatry 33:925–933, 1992

Leonard HL, Lenane MC, Swedo SE, et al: A double-blind comparison of clomipramine and desipramine treatment of severe onychophagia (nail biting). Arch Gen Psychiatry 48:821–827, 1991

Lewis MH, Bodfish JW, Powell SB, et al: Clomipramine treatment for self-injurious behavior of individuals with mental retardation: a double-blind comparison with placebo. Am J Ment Retard 100:654–665, 1996

Lochner C, Stein DJ: Obsessive-compulsive spectrum disorders in obsessive-compulsive disorder and other anxiety disorders. Psychopathology 43:389–396, 2010

Lochner C, du Toit PL, Zungu-Dirwayi N, et al: Childhood trauma in obsessive-compulsive disorder, trichotillomania, and controls. Depress Anxiety 15:66–68, 2002

Lochner C, Hemmings SMJ, Kinnear CJ, et al: Cluster analysis of obsessive-compulsive spectrum disorders in patients with obsessive-compulsive disorder: clinical and genetic correlates. Compr Psychiatry 46:14–19, 2005

MacLean PD: A Triune Concept of the Brain and Behavior. Toronto, ON, Canada, University of Toronto Press, 1973

Martin A, Pigott TA, Lalonde FM, et al: Lack of evidence for Huntington's disease–like cognitive dysfunction in obsessive-compulsive disorder. Biol Psychiatry 33:345–353, 1993

Martin A, Scahill L, Vitulano L, et al: Stimulant use and trichotillomania. J Am Acad Child Adolesc Psychiatry 37:349–350, 1998

Martin LJ, Spicer DM, Lewis MH, et al: Social deprivation of infant rhesus monkeys alters the chemoarchitecture of the brain, I: subcortical regions. J Neurosci 11:3344–3358, 1991

McGrath CM, Kennedy RE, Hoye W, et al: Stereotypic movement disorder after acquired brain injury. Brain Inj 16:447–451, 2002

Ninan PT, Rothbaum BO, Stipetic M, et al: CSF 5-HIAA as a predictor of treatment response in trichotillomania. Psychopharmacol Bull 28:451–455, 1992

Novak CE, Keuthen NJ, Stewart SE, et al: A twin concordance study of trichotillomania. Am J Med Genet B Neuropsychiatr Genet 150B:944–949, 2009

Odlaug BL, Chamberlain SR, Grant JE: Motor inhibition and cognitive flexibility in pathologic skin picking. Prog Neuropsychopharmacol Biol Psychiatry 34:208–211, 2010

O'Sullivan RL, Rauch SL, Breiter HC, et al: Reduced basal ganglia volumes in trichotillomania measured via morphometric magnetic resonance imaging. Biol Psychiatry 42:39–45, 1997

O'Sullivan RL, Lipper G, Lerner EA: The neuro-immuno-cutaneous-endocrine network: relationship of mind and skin. Arch Dermatol 134:1431–1435, 1998

O'Sullivan R, Christenson GA, Stein DJ: Pharmacotherapy of trichotillomania, in Trichotillomania. Edited by Stein DJ, Christenson GA, Hollander E. Washington, DC, American Psychiatric Press, 1999, pp 93–123

Rapoport JL, Ryland DH, Kriete M: Drug treatment of canine acral lick. Arch Gen Psychiatry 48:517–521, 1992

Rauch SL, Wright CI, Savage CR, et al: Brain activation during implicit sequence learning in individuals with trichotillomania. Psychiatry Res 154:233–240, 2007

Reinhardt V: Hair pulling: a review. Lab Anim 39:361–369, 2005

Rettew DC, Cheslow DL, Rapoport JL, et al: Neuropsychological test-performance in trichotillomania: a further link with obsessive-compulsive disorder. J Anxiety Disord 5:225–235, 1991

Richter MA, Summerfeldt LJ, Antony MM, et al: Obsessive-compulsive spectrum conditions in obsessive-compulsive disorder and other anxiety disorders. Depress Anxiety 18:118–127, 2003

Ridley RM: The psychology of perseverative and stereotyped behavior. Prog Neurobiol 44:221–231, 1994

Schroeder SR, Oster-Granite ML, Berkson G, et al: Self-injurious behavior: gene-brain-behavior relationships. Ment Retard Dev Disabil Res Rev 7:3–12, 2001

Schroeder SR, Loupe PS, Tessel RE: Animal models of self-injurious behavior: induction, prevention, and recovery. Int Rev Res Ment Retard 36:195–231, 2008

Seibert LM, Crowell-Davis SL, Wilson GH, et al: Placebo-controlled clomipramine trial for the treatment of feather picking disorder in cockatoos. J Am Anim Hosp Assoc 40:261–269, 2004

Stanley MA, Hannay HJ, Breckenridge JK: The neuropsychology of trichotillomania. J Anxiety Disord 11:473–488, 1997

Stein DJ: Neurobiology of the obsessive-compulsive spectrum disorders. Biol Psychiatry 47:296–304, 2000

Stein DJ, Hollander E: Low-dose pimozide augmentation of serotonin reuptake blockers in the treatment of trichotillomania. J Clin Psychiatry 53:123–126, 1992

Stein DJ, Lochner C: Obsessive-compulsive spectrum disorders: a multidimensional approach. Psychiatr Clin North Am 29:343–351, 2006

Stein DJ, Simeon D: Pharmacotherapy of stereotypic movement disorders. Psychiatr Ann 28:327–334, 1998

Stein DJ, Dodman NH, Borchelt P, et al: Behavioral disorders in veterinary practice: relevance to psychiatry. Compr Psychiatry 35:275–285, 1994a

Stein DJ, Hollander E, Simeon D, et al: Neurological soft signs in female patients with trichotillomania. J Neuropsychiatry Clin Neurosci 6:184–187, 1994b

Stein DJ, Hollander E, Cohen L, et al: Serotonergic responsivity in trichotillomania: neuroendocrine effects of m-chlorophenylpiperazine. Biol Psychiatry 37:414–416, 1995

Stein DJ, Coetzer R, Lee M, et al: Magnetic resonance brain imaging in women with obsessive-compulsive disorder and trichotillomania. Psychiatry Res 74:177–182, 1997a

Stein DJ, Wessels C, Carr J, et al: Hair pulling in a patient with Sydenham's chorea. Am J Psychiatry 154:1320, 1997b

Stein DJ, Mendelsohn I, Potocnik F, et al: Use of the selective serotonin reuptake inhibitor citalopram in a possible animal analogue of obsessive-compulsive disorder. Depress Anxiety 8:39–42, 1998

Stein DJ, Goodman WK, Rauch SL: The cognitive-affective neuroscience of obsessive-compulsive disorder. Curr Psychiatry Rep 2:341–346, 2000

Stein DJ, van Heerden B, Hugo C, et al: Functional brain imaging and pharmacotherapy in trichotillomania: single photon emission computed tomography before and after treatment with the selective serotonin reuptake inhibitor citalopram. Prog Neuropsychopharmacol Biol Psychiatry 26:885–890, 2002

Stein DJ, Chamberlain SR, Fineberg N: An A-B-C model of habit disorders: hair-pulling, skin-picking, and other stereotypic conditions. CNS Spectr 11:824–827, 2006

Swedo SE: A double-blind comparison of clomipramine and desipramine in the treatment of trichotillomania (hair pulling). N Engl J Med 321:497–501, 1989

Swedo SE, Rapoport JL, Leonard HL, et al: Regional cerebral glucose metabolism of women with trichotillomania. Arch Gen Psychiatry 48:828–833, 1991

Symons FJ, Thompson A, Rodriguez MC: Self-injurious behavior and the efficacy of naltrexone treatment: a quantitative synthesis. Ment Retard Dev Disabil Res Rev 10:193–200, 2004

Van Ameringen M, Mancini C, Oakman JM, et al: The potential role of haloperidol in the treatment of trichotillomania. J Affect Disord 56:219–226, 1999

Van Ameringen M, Mancini C, Patterson B, et al: A randomized placebo controlled trial of olanzapine in trichotillomania. Eur Neuropsychopharmacol 16:S452, 2006

Vythilingum B, Warwick J, van Kradenburg J, et al: SPECT scans in identical twins with trichotillomania. J Neuropsychiatry Clin Neurosci 14:340–342, 2002

Welch JM, Lu J, Rodriguiz RM, et al: Cortico-striatal synaptic defects and OCD-like behaviours in Sapap3-mutant mice. Nature 448:894–900, 2007

Zuchner S, Cuccaro ML, Tran-Viet KN, et al: SLITRK1 mutations in trichotillomania. Mol Psychiatry 11:888–889, 2006

Zuchner S, Wendland JR, Ashley-Koch AE, et al: Multiple rare SAPAP3 missense variants in trichotillomania and OCD. Mol Psychiatry 14:6–9, 2009

Part 2

DIAGNOSIS AND
EVALUATION

Chapter 5

DIAGNOSIS AND COMORBIDITY

Christopher A. Flessner, Ph.D.

Aside from trichotillomania, a distinct diagnostic category does not exist for skin picking or other stereotypic disorders such as nail biting, teeth grinding, head banging, thumb sucking, and body rocking. This chapter is intended to provide a useful reference for practitioners unfamiliar with the diagnosis, patterns of comorbidity, and differential diagnoses present among individuals exhibiting symptoms of these disorders. The aim of this chapter is threefold. First, I intend to provide a useful approach to the diagnosis of these disorders. Second, I offer data regarding patterns of comorbidity typical among these populations. Finally, I describe important factors to consider in the differential diagnosis of each disorder. Before we begin, however, I would like to offer a word of caution to those who may be less familiar with these disorders. Although substantial overlap exists between trichotillomania, skin picking, and other stereotypic disorders, as is highlighted throughout this clinical manual, each has unique facets (e.g., approaches to diagnosis, differentiation from other disorders). Therefore, it would be unwise for practitioners to assume "one size fits all." Careful attention to differential diagnoses germane to these respective disorders, in particular, can yield critically important information beneficial to the treatment process and ultimately treatment outcome. Please keep this fact in mind as you read this chapter.

TRICHOTILLOMANIA

Diagnosis

Trichotillomania is presently classified as an impulse-control disorder (ICD; code 312.39) in DSM-IV-TR (American Psychiatric Association 2000). It is characterized by the recurrent pulling out of one's hair, resulting in noticeable hair loss (Criterion A). Although it may seem counterintuitive, it is often not a simple task to identify "noticeable hair loss." This may be particularly true for practitioners less familiar with trichotillomania. Patients often wear wigs, other accessories (i.e., hats, scarves), or cosmetics to hide their hair loss. Therefore, it is important to consider whether, in the absence of attempts to cover or hide pulling, hair loss is noticeable upon inspection. Practitioners should make every effort (when possible, of course) to examine the area(s) from which the patient reports pulling. Depending on the patient's level of comfort and the rapport that has been established, this may be a task that is most appropriate for the end of an initial session or perhaps for a second meeting.

Although hair pulling is the trademark symptom of trichotillomania, pulling must also be accompanied by an increasing sense of tension prior to or while attempting to resist pulling (Criterion B) *and* a feeling of gratification, relief, or pleasure after pulling (Criterion C). Practitioners may be best served by developing a battery of synonyms for *tension, relief, gratification,* and *pleasure* to use with patients who are unable to firmly grasp the message or underlying meaning of Criteria B and C. This may be particularly true for children. In fact, many clinical researchers choose to confer a diagnosis of trichotillomania in the absence of reported tension prior to and/or relief after pulling (Diefenbach et al. 2005; Watson and Allen 1993; Watson et al. 2000). Therefore, the absence of Criteria B and C should not automatically discount a diagnosis of trichotillomania. Finally, hair pulling must cause clinically significant impairment or distress in day-to-day functioning (e.g., social, interpersonal, academic, or occupational) (Franklin et al. 2008; Woods et al. 2006a) and must not be better accounted for by another mental health condition (American Psychiatric Association 2000).

Common Comorbidities

A variety of psychiatric diagnoses have been found comorbid with trichotillomania. As many as 57% of adults with trichotillomania have a comorbid diagnosis, most commonly mood and anxiety disorders (Christenson et al. 1991; Diefenbach et al. 2002; Schlosser et al. 1994; Woods et al. 2006b). Recently, Woods et al. (2006b) found that major depression (28.6%) and obsessive-compulsive disorder (OCD; 10.7%) were the most common comorbid disorders among a treatment-seeking sample of adults with trichotillomania. Similarly, a recent large-scale, Internet-based study found that 34% of adults who had symptoms corresponding with a trichotillomania diagnosis reported seeking help for a psychosocial problem other than trichotillomania, with mood (e.g., depression, bipolar disorder) and anxiety (e.g., OCD, social phobia, agoraphobia) disorders among the most common concerns (Woods et al. 2006b).

Scant research has examined comorbid diagnoses among children with trichotillomania. Early research suggested that about 70% of these children met diagnostic criteria for at least one other psychiatric diagnosis (Reeve et al. 1992), with anxiety and mood disorders representing the most likely diagnoses (King et al. 1995). However, a more recent study involving a treatment-seeking sample found that 39.1% of children with trichotillomania presented with a comorbid diagnosis. Of these children with a comorbid diagnosis, 30.4% and 10.9% presented with an anxiety or an externalizing disorder, respectively (Tolin et al. 2007). Within these respective domains, generalized anxiety (13.0%), social phobia (8.7%), OCD (6.5%), attention-deficit/hyperactivity disorder (ADHD; 8.7%), and oppositional defiant disorder (ODD; 6.5%) were among the most common diagnoses. Similarly, a recent Internet-based study found that 38.3% of children had been diagnosed with at least one other mental health disorder. Among these diagnoses, anxiety disorders (24.1%), mood disorders (18.8%), and ADHD (16.5%) were the most common (Franklin et al. 2008). Collectively, more recent evidence appears to suggest that comorbid diagnoses, particularly anxiety, mood, and disruptive behavior disorders, are common among children with trichotillomania, although perhaps not occurring as often as was once believed.

Although pulling at a young age may simply be a benign habit (Friman et al. 1992), psychiatric comorbidity is evident in even younger children (<3 years of age). At least one study found that 50% of toddlers who pulled their hair met requirements for a comorbid anxiety disorder, 40% displayed developmental problems, 20% had chronic pediatric concerns, and 100% of the sample had family stressors such as parental separation, homelessness, unemployment, or parent mental illness (Wright and Holmes 2003). Very little research, however, exists among this younger population. Therefore, careful assessment and caution are necessary when working with these young children. Collectively, findings from the trichotillomania literature suggest that a variety of comorbid diagnoses are present among young and older children and adults with trichotillomania. This evidence can help practitioners and researchers develop a better understanding of disorders to be ruled out in the differential diagnosis before conferring a trichotillomania diagnosis.

Differential Diagnosis

Ruling out other possible diagnoses is a core diagnostic criterion of trichotillomania (American Psychiatric Association 2000). It is important to understand, however, that it is not uncommon for children, in particular, or adults to deny hair pulling or report a lack of pulling awareness. This denial of or lack of awareness is most often *but not always* attributed to what has been termed *automatic* pulling—that is, pulling that occurs outside of one's awareness, such as while reading, watching television, or lying in bed (Flessner et al. 2007, 2008). Therefore, practitioners must assess whether hair loss/hair pulling may be due to a general medical condition (e.g., dry scalp or skin, dermatological condition). For example, DSM-IV-TR provides a comprehensive list of additional medical explanations for hair loss (alopecia) that must be ruled out before a diagnosis of trichotillomania can be conferred, including alopecia areata, male pattern baldness, chronic discoid lupus erythematosus, lichen planopilaris, folliculitis decalvans, pseudopelade, and alopecia mucinosa (American Psychiatric Association 2000). In addition, a patient with chronically dry scalp may pull to alleviate an itching sensation rather than as the result of an underlying tension. Consultation with the patient's pediatrician, dermatologist, or primary care physician may be necessary to formally rule out these potential medical explanations for hair loss.

Individuals with trichotillomania present with a variety of comorbid psychiatric conditions. Therefore, it is of great importance that practitioners assess whether the patient's hair pulling is solely attributed to trichotillomania or is better characterized as symptomatic of some other disorder. For example, a diagnosis of trichotillomania should not be conferred if pulling occurs in response to delusions or hallucinations (e.g., pulling because the patient believes bugs are crawling on him or her), which is characteristic of schizophrenia or related psychotic disorder. However, perhaps the two most common diagnoses to consider in the differential diagnosis of trichotillomania are OCD and body dysmorphic disorder (BDD).

Clinical researchers have begun to classify trichotillomania as part of an obsessive-compulsive spectrum of disorders (Bartz and Hollander 2006; Flessner et al. 2009) because of similar elevations in anxiety prior to many pulling episodes and decreases in anxiety subsequent to pulling. Trichotillomania differs from OCD, however, in that the compulsions associated with trichotillomania are specific to hair pulling. The "obsessions" most often seen among those with trichotillomania are often characteristic of the worries and thoughts common to "focused" pulling (see Chapter 1, "Trichotillomania: Epidemiology and Clinical Characteristics"). If obsessions about other aspects of the individual's life and compulsions that are not specific to hair pulling are present, diagnoses of both trichotillomania and OCD may be appropriate. Similarly, ambiguity exists in differentiating trichotillomania from BDD. Given the primary symptom of trichotillomania (i.e., recurrent hair pulling), it is not surprising that individuals become overly distressed by their appearance. However, individuals with BDD are frequently overly distressed about a variety of aspects to their appearance, not solely hair loss. In fact, adults with trichotillomania tend to experience worries and thoughts about their pulling that are often not present among those with BDD (Allen and Hollander 2004). Unfortunately, there is a general lack of research with regard to behaviors differentiating trichotillomania from either OCD or BDD among children. Therefore, clinicians must exercise considerable caution and conduct a thorough functional assessment prior to conferring any of these diagnoses upon patients, especially children.

SKIN PICKING

Diagnosis

Skin picking has no specific diagnostic classification in DSM-IV-TR. Most often, however, it is classified as either a stereotypic movement disorder (SMD) or an impulse-control disorder not otherwise specified (ICD-NOS). As may be inferred, then, detailing precise diagnostic criteria for skin picking is difficult. For example, ICD-NOS provides a broad classification reserved for behaviors that demonstrate a lack of impulse control yet are not better accounted for by another psychiatric condition. In fact, many view skin picking and trichotillomania as topographically different yet functionally similar (i.e., different on the outside, similar on the inside; see "Common Comorbidities" section that follows). As in trichotillomania, individuals who pick their skin frequently employ strategies such as the use of makeup, specific hairstyles, or clothing (e.g., long sleeves, pants) to conceal the effects of their behavior (Flessner and Woods 2006), thus making the diagnostic process less straightforward. As such, practitioners more comfortable with the use of an ICD-NOS label for skin-picking patients are advised to substitute skin picking for hair pulling in the diagnostic criteria described earlier for trichotillomania. Consequently, strategies used for the diagnosis of an individual with trichotillomania will likely also be of great benefit for diagnosing skin-picking disorder as well.

SMD provides a narrower classification and requires that the patient fulfill several diagnostic criteria. First, the patient must engage in a repetitive, seemingly driven, and nonfunctional motor behavior (Criterion A; e.g., skin picking) for at least 4 weeks (Criterion F). It is often helpful to provide patients with a timeline or anchor event to adequately assess duration. For example, asking the patient whether picking began before or after a recent holiday, birthday, or some other significant event may be helpful in pinpointing a more precise timeline for the behavior. In addition, skin picking must markedly interfere with normal activities (e.g., causes patient to be late for school, work, or appointments; increases social distance from peers) or result in self-inflicted bodily injury requiring medical treatment (Criterion B). If mental retardation is present, skin picking must be severe enough to become the focus of treatment (Criterion C). The behavior must also not be better accounted for by the physiological effects of a substance or medical condition (Criterion E). Similar to the strategy employed earlier for assessing onset and duration of skin picking, practitioners are advised to develop a detailed timeline regarding the onset of the patient's skin picking and any illicit or non-illicit drug use that may coincide with and perhaps better account for the patient's symptoms (see "Differential Diagnosis" section that follows). Skin picking must also not be better described by symptoms attributed to another psychiatric condition (e.g., BDD, pervasive developmental disorders; Criterion D). Because skin picking results in damage to one's body, the specifier "with self-injurious behavior" may be appropriate for patients exhibiting this behavior.

This description suggests that clinicians can choose the diagnostic classification that they feel fits their patient best. However, it is important to note that most clinical researchers believe that only two primary criteria need to be present (at least for the purposes of research) to confer a diagnosis of skin-picking disorder: 1) recurrent picking of the skin accompanied by visible tissue damage and 2) clinically significant distress and/or functional impairment as a result of the picking (Bohne et al. 2002; Keuthen et al. 2000; Teng et al. 2002; Wilhelm et al. 1999). It is also important to consider whether skin picking occurs independent of or in conjunction with another psychiatric condition. Because of this fairly consistent approach to the diagnosis of skin-picking disorder, these diagnostic criteria will largely guide the discussion of comorbid diagnoses.

Common Comorbidities

A small but growing body of literature has examined comorbid psychiatric diagnoses among those who pick their skin. However, it should be noted that this literature is almost entirely limited to adult populations. Therefore, data presented in the following discussion are limited to adult samples. A variety of psychiatric conditions have been found comorbid with skin picking. A recent study by Odlaug and Grant (2008b) found that 54.5% of adults with skin-picking disorder have a lifetime history of any comorbid diagnosis. This rate is remarkably similar to the relative prevalence of comorbidities found among those with trichotillomania (i.e., ~57%; see earlier discussion).

Earlier in this section, I suggested that the terms *hair pulling* and *skin picking* could be interchanged with relative ease for clinicians seeking to confer an ICD-NOS diagnosis on an individual who picks his or her skin. Research consistently demonstrates a great degree of overlap between trichotillomania and skin-picking disorder (Lochner et al. 2002; Odlaug and Grant 2008a,

2008b). As a result, research studies frequently place individuals with skin picking or hair pulling into the same group, often referred to as "grooming conditions," for the purpose of analyzing data (Flessner et al. 2009; Grant and Christenson 2007; Hanna et al. 2005). Recent findings also suggest that compulsive nail biting occurs at similarly high rates among individuals with skin picking or hair pulling (i.e., 25% and 21.2%, respectively; Odlaug and Grant 2008a). Perhaps not surprisingly then, Odlaug and Grant (2008b) found that 38.3% of adults with skin-picking disorder demonstrated a lifetime diagnosis of trichotillomania. Previous studies have demonstrated similarly elevated rates of trichotillomania among those with skin-picking disorder (Wilhelm et al. 1999). As such, it is important for practitioners to understand and assess for the presence of both trichotillomania and skin picking among those presenting with either concern.

Adults who pick their skin present with a variety of other comorbid diagnoses. Common comorbid diagnoses among adults with skin-picking disorder include major depressive disorder (MDD), nail biting, OCD, and mild to moderate levels of anxiety (Bloch et al. 2001; Odlaug and Grant 2008a, 2008b; Simeon et al. 1997; Wilhelm et al. 1999). Wilhelm et al. (1999) found that 52% of adults who picked their skin met diagnostic criteria for OCD, 39% for alcohol abuse/dependence, 26% for MDD, 26% for illicit drug abuse/dependence, 23% for dysthymia, and 23% for social phobia. More recent research, however, has generally found lower rates of these comorbid diagnoses. Odlaug and Grant (2008a) evaluated 60 adults with a primary diagnosis of skin-picking disorder and found that nearly 17% met diagnostic criteria for OCD in their lifetime, 3.3% for any substance use disorder, 31.7% for MDD, and 3.3% for social phobia. Other recent research has found similar rates of comorbid diagnoses. Discrepancies in comorbidity rates among these studies are likely due to differences in research methodology. Wilhelm et al. (1999) recruited adults who picked their skin regardless of whether skin picking was the primary diagnosis or secondary to another condition. Conversely, Odlaug and Grant (2008a) examined only adults with a primary diagnosis of skin-picking disorder. As such, more recent findings (e.g., Odlaug and Grant 2008a) may be more indicative of the actual clinical presentation of adults with a primary diagnosis of skin-picking disorder.

Differential Diagnosis

Akin to a thorough diagnostic evaluation for trichotillomania, practitioners must assess whether skin picking is the result of a general medical condition (e.g., dry skin, dermatological condition) or, in the case of an ICD-NOS diagnosis, in response to an increasing sense of tension prior to picking. However, skin picking may also develop as the result of cocaine, methylphenidate, phenelzine, amphetamine, anticholinergic, or other substance use/abuse (Bishop 1983; Denys et al. 2003). As a result, the timeline described previously can be helpful for differentiating whether skin picking occurs independent of or as a result of substance use/abuse. Because of this interesting relationship between the occurrence of skin picking and possible substance use/abuse, it can be helpful for practitioners and researchers to consult with colleagues in related fields (e.g., psychiatry, primary care, substance use/abuse counseling) before dismissing the possible deleterious effects of even commonly prescribed psychotropic medication(s).

As alluded to in the preceding paragraph, practitioners must assess whether the skin picking occurs independent or is symptomatic of another psychiatric condition. For example, it is important to consider whether skin picking occurs in response to delusional symptoms characteristic of a psychotic disorder. As is described in greater detail later (see "Other Stereotypic Disorders"), skin picking and other stereotypic disorders (e.g., SMDs) frequently occur in the presence of mental retardation or pervasive developmental disorders. If this is the case, practitioners must ensure that skin picking is not better attributed to these conditions. Differentiation should also be made between skin picking and OCD—that is, are obsessions specific only to skin picking, or do they occur in other aspects of an individual's life as well? However, what is perhaps most important in the differential diagnosis is to distinguish skin picking alone from skin picking that is symptomatic of BDD.

The prevalence of skin picking among adults (primarily women) diagnosed with BDD is quite high. A recent study found that 44.9% of adults with BDD reported a lifetime occurrence of skin picking (Grant et al. 2006). Conversely, Odlaug and Grant (2008a) found that among adults with a primary diagnosis of skin-picking disorder only, 5% met diagnostic criteria for BDD in their lifetime. These findings highlight the importance of distinguishing between skin picking that may be worthy of treatment by itself and skin picking that is symptomatic of BDD. By definition, skin picking results in some degree (ranging from mild to very severe) of physical defect to one's skin. However, picking that is secondary to BDD is often in an attempt to eliminate some perceived blemish or imperfection to one's skin rather than the result of some underlying tension or stereotypic behavior. As a result, it is important for practitioners treating individuals who pick their skin to conduct a thorough functional assessment to better delineate the proper diagnosis to confer. The subsequent intervention, whether behavioral or pharmacological, will likely differ to a great extent depending upon the results of this assessment.

OTHER STEREOTYPIC DISORDERS

Diagnosis

Other stereotypic disorders include a variety of repetitive behaviors, including teeth grinding (bruxism), mouth chewing, lip biting, thumb sucking, body rocking, head banging, and nail biting. As with skin picking, no specific diagnostic criteria exist for these behaviors. In turn, SMD is the most often used diagnostic category for this class of repetitive behaviors. From this point forward, SMD is used to refer to a diagnosis conferred on individuals presenting with these behaviors.

In an attempt to provide a set of criteria that may be more easily assessable in clinical practice, researchers often employ a hybrid approach to classification, requiring that the individual engage in the behavior of interest (e.g., nail biting, teeth grinding) at least five times per day for at least 4 weeks and that the behavior cause functional or physical damage or impairment (e.g., bleeding, sores, interference at work or school; Teng et al. 2002). Importantly, some of these repetitive behaviors (e.g., nail biting, teeth grinding, head banging) are likely to cause physical damage to one's body. In cases such as this (similar to skin picking), the specifier "with self-injurious behavior" may be appropriate, whereas for other behaviors (e.g., thumb sucking, body rocking) this specification may not be appropriate. In summary, the approaches for conferring a diagnosis of SMD upon an individual with skin picking or some other repetitive behavior (i.e., other stereotypic disorder) are remarkably similar. However, it is of great importance to understand the limited research examining comorbid psychiatric diagnoses and, in turn, differential diagnosis among children and adults presenting with these other stereotypic disorders.

Common Comorbidities

A substantial body of literature exists demonstrating the frequency with which repetitive behaviors are present in individuals diagnosed with mental retardation or a pervasive developmental disorder (i.e., autism, Asperger's, Rett syndrome; Long and Miltenberger 1998; Matson et al. 2009; Mooney et al. 2009). In this literature, these repetitive behaviors are often referred to as *stereotypies*. The confirmation of an SMD diagnosis, however, requires that the repetitive behavior of interest (e.g., body rocking) not be better accounted for by a pervasive developmental disorder (see "Differential Diagnosis"). Although it is important for practitioners to be aware of these apparently high rates of comorbidity, this overlap does not suggest that patients presenting with such stereotypies will necessarily meet diagnostic criteria for an SMD. In fact, in many instances this will not be the case. For example, one study found that the repetitive behaviors reported by nearly 62% of adults were better accounted for by another Axis I disorder (Castellanos et al. 1996). I use the term *repetitive behaviors*, as opposed to *stereotypies*, to refer to those behaviors that are *not* better accounted for by a pervasive developmental disorder. In turn, it is important to understand the patterns of comorbidity among typically developing individuals who may indeed qualify for an SMD diagnosis and exhibit any of the myriad repetitive behaviors described earlier.

Repetitive behaviors are a frequent occurrence among typically developing children and adults. These individuals may also present with various comorbid psychiatric concerns. Perhaps because of the perceived benign nature of these repetitive behaviors, however, few studies have conducted comprehensive diagnostic evaluations of individuals presenting with these concerns. Rafaeli-Mor et al. (1999) examined college students who engaged in body rocking and found that 14.7% met diagnostic criteria for generalized anxiety disorder, 13.2% for MDD, 7.4% for specific phobia, 6.0% for dysthymia, and 5.9% for social phobia. Conversely, Castellanos et al. (1996) found that 92% of adults meeting diagnostic criteria for an SMD (e.g., body rocking, thumb sucking) also met diagnostic criteria for an affective or anxiety disorder during their lifetime. Most recently, Ghanizadeh (2008) found that 14% of consecutive referrals to a child and adolescent psychiatry clinic engaged in nail biting. Although not surprising given the site from which the children were recruited, 93.6% met diagnostic criteria for another disorder. Of these, 74.6% met diagnostic criteria for ADHD, 36% for ODD, 20.6% for separation anxiety, 15.6% for enuresis, 12.7% for a tic disorder, and 11.1% for OCD. Excluding those who pulled their hair (11.1%), 54% also engaged in at least one other repetitive behavior (i.e., lip biting, teeth grinding, head banging, or skin picking). Although limited in scope, these findings suggest that individuals presenting with other stereotypic disorders (i.e., SMDs) also present with a variety of comorbid diagnoses, in particular anxiety and mood disorders. However, findings by Castellanos et al. (1996) also clearly suggest that other diagnoses should be considered before conferring an SMD diagnosis.

Differential Diagnosis

The differential diagnosis employed for skin picking resembles in some ways that for other SMDs. Practitioners must assess whether these repetitive behaviors are the result of a general medical condition, substance use/abuse, or another psychiatric disorder (i.e., delusions/hallucination associated with a psychotic disorder, compulsions associated with OCD). Individuals who pull their hair but do not engage in any other repetitive behavior are not eligible for an SMD diagnosis. However, as described previously, trichotillomania and other repetitive behaviors often co-occur (i.e., skin picking, nail biting).

As a result, it is not uncommon for individuals who pull their hair and, for example, pick their skin to receive both a trichotillomania and an SMD diagnosis. Practitioners must also be aware of several additional psychiatric conditions in particular that must be ruled out before conferring an SMD diagnosis on individuals presenting with these repetitive behaviors.

An SMD diagnosis cannot be conferred if the repetitive behavior (e.g., body rocking, head banging) is better accounted for by a pervasive developmental disorder. As such, a careful diagnostic assessment and evaluation is necessary to formally rule out these potential alternative diagnoses (i.e., autism, Prader-Willi syndrome, or Rett syndrome). Conversely, a diagnosis of SMD can be conferred among individuals diagnosed with mental retardation *only* if the repetitive behavior is of sufficient severity to dictate that the behavior be the focus of treatment. If this is not the case, SMD should not be diagnosed. As such, clinical judgment will play a large role in determining whether both the SMD *and* mental retardation diagnoses are appropriate, rather than simply the latter.

SMDs are often misdiagnosed as complex tics characteristic of a tic disorder (Singer 2009). However, several important features differentiate these disorders. First, the pattern of repetitive behaviors characteristic of an SMD is often fixed, with little fluctuation over time, whereas tics frequently change (i.e., new ones develop, old ones fade away). Second, although not the case for all SMDs (i.e., skin picking), these repetitive behaviors are rarely preceded by a premonitory urge or sensation as is characteristic of tics (Woods et al. 2005). That is, children (>10 years of age) and adults with simple or complex tics often report an internal sensation prior to engaging in a tic (e.g., tickle in throat before a throat-clearing tic, tingle in the back of eyes before an eye-blinking tic). This is not the case for most SMDs. Finally, as Singer (2009) highlights, stereotypic/repetitive behaviors most often involve the arms, hands, or entire body. Conversely, although tics may occur in these bodily locations, tics are more commonly associated with the eyes, face, head, and shoulders. None of these rules by themselves are sufficient to differentiate a complex tic from a repetitive behavior characteristic of SMD. However, collectively, they provide a reliable means of differentiating the behaviors characteristic of these disorders.

CONCLUSION

The decision rules provided throughout this chapter are designed to be helpful for practitioners caring for patients presenting with these various repetitive behaviors. It is my hope that many of the techniques and strategies suggested herein are well within the capabilities of most seasoned practitioners. For those practitioners less accustomed to working with these populations, however, the preceding and subsequent chapters in this clinical manual will provide the necessary background for adequately addressing concerns related to the diagnosis and differential diagnosis of trichotillomania, skin picking, and other stereotypic disorders. What is more, as with any patient presenting with a complex psychiatric concern, consultation with other colleagues is always recommended.

REFERENCES

Allen A, Hollander E: Similarities and differences between body dysmorphic disorder and other disorders. Psychiatr Ann 34:927–933, 2004

American Psychiatric Association: Diagnostic and Statistical Manual of Mental Disorders, 4th Edition, Text Revision. Washington, DC, American Psychiatric Association, 2000

Bartz JA, Hollander E: Is obsessive-compulsive disorder an anxiety disorder? Prog Neuropsychopharmacol Biol Psychiatry 30:338–352, 2006

Bishop ER Jr: Monosymptomatic hypochondriacal syndromes in dermatology. J Am Acad Dermatol 9:152–158, 1983

Bloch MR, Elliott M, Thompson H, et al: Fluoxetine in pathologic skin-picking: open-label and double-blind results. Psychosomatics 42:314–319, 2001

Bohne A, Wilhelm S, Keuthen NJ, et al: Skin picking in German students: prevalence, phenomenology, and associated characteristics. Behav Modif 26:320–339, 2002

Castellanos FX, Ritchie GF, Marsh WL, et al: DSM-IV stereotypic movement disorder: persistence of stereotypies of infancy in intellectually normal adolescents and adults. J Clin Psychiatry 57:116–122, 1996

Christenson GA, Mackenzie TB, Mitchell JE: Characteristics of 60 adult chronic hair pullers. Am J Psychiatry 148:365–370, 1991

Denys D, van Megen HJ, Westenberg HG: Emerging skin-picking behaviour after serotonin reuptake inhibitor–treatment in patients with obsessive-compulsive disorder: possible mechanisms and implications for clinical care. J Psychopharmacol 17:127–129, 2003

Diefenbach GJ, Mouton-Odum S, Stanley MA: Affective correlates of trichotillomania. Behav Res Ther 40:1305–1315, 2002

Diefenbach GJ, Tolin DF, Hannan S, et al: Trichotillomania: impact on psychosocial functioning and quality of life. Behav Res Ther 43:869–884, 2005

Flessner CA, Woods DW: Phenomenological characteristics, social problems, and the economic impact associated with chronic skin picking. Behav Modif 30:944–963, 2006

Flessner CA, Woods DW, Franklin ME, et al: The Milwaukee Inventory for Styles of Trichotillomania–Child Version (MIST-C): initial development and psychometric properties. Behav Modif 31:896–918, 2007

Flessner CA, Conelea CA, Woods DW, et al: Styles of pulling in trichotillomania: exploring differences in symptom severity, phenomenology, and functional impact. Behav Res Ther 46:345–357, 2008

Flessner CA, Berman N, Garcia A, et al: Symptom profiles in pediatric obsessive-compulsive disorder (OCD): the effects of comorbid grooming conditions. J Anxiety Disord 23:753–759, 2009

Franklin M, Flessner CA, Woods DW, et al: The Child and Adolescent Trichotillomania Impact Project: descriptive psychopathology, comorbidity, functional impairment, and treatment utilization. J Dev Behav Pediatr 29:493–500, 2008

Friman PC, Blum NJ, Rostain A: Is hair pulling benign? J Am Acad Child Adolesc Psychiatry 31:991–992, 1992

Ghanizadeh A: Association of nail biting and psychiatric disorders in children and their parents in a psychiatrically referred sample of children. Child Adolesc Psychiatry Ment Health 2:13, 2008

Grant JE, Christenson GA: Examination of gender in pathologic grooming behaviors. Psychiatr Q 78:259–267, 2007

Grant JE, Menard W, Phillips KA: Pathological skin picking in individuals with body dysmorphic disorder. Gen Hosp Psychiatry 28:487–493, 2006

Hanna GL, Fischer D, Chadha K, et al: Familial and sporadic subtypes of early onset obsessive-compulsive disorder. Biol Psychiatry 57:895–900, 2005

Keuthen NJ, Deckersbach T, Wilhelm S, et al: Repetitive skin-picking in a student population and comparison with a sample of self-injurious skin-pickers. Psychosomatics 41:210–215, 2000

King RA, Scahill L, Vitulano LA, et al: Childhood trichotillomania: clinical phenomenology, comorbidity, and family genetics. J Am Acad Child Adolesc Psychiatry 34:1451–1459, 1995

Lochner C, Simeon D, Niehaus DJ, et al: Trichotillomania and skin-picking: a phenomenological comparison. Depress Anxiety 15:83–86, 2002

Long ES, Miltenberger RG: A review of behavioral and pharmacological treatments for habit disorders in individuals with mental retardation. J Behav Ther Exp Psychiatry 29:143–156, 1998

Matson JL, Dempsey T, Fodstad JC: Stereotypies and repetitive/restrictive behaviours in infants with autism and pervasive developmental disorder. Dev Neurorehabil 12:122–127, 2009

Mooney EL, Gray KM, Tonge BJ, et al: Factor analytic study of repetitive behaviours in young children with pervasive developmental disorders. J Autism Dev Disord 39:765–774, 2009

Odlaug BL, Grant JE: Clinical characteristics and medical complications of pathologic skin picking. Gen Hosp Psychiatry 30:61–66, 2008a

Odlaug BL, Grant JE: Trichotillomania and pathologic skin picking: clinical comparison with an examination of comorbidity. Ann Clin Psychiatry 20:57–63, 2008b

Rafaeli-Mor N, Foster L, Berkson G: Self-reported body-rocking and other habits in college students. Am J Ment Retard 104:1–10, 1999

Reeve EA, Bernstein GA, Christenson GA: Clinical characteristics and psychiatric comorbidity in children with trichotillomania. J Am Acad Child Adolesc Psychiatry 31:132–138, 1992

Schlosser S, Black DW, Blum N, et al: The demography, phenomenology, and family history of 22 persons with compulsive hair pulling. Ann Clin Psychiatry 6:147–152, 1994

Simeon D, Stein DJ, Gross S, et al: A double-blind trial of fluoxetine in pathologic skin picking. J Clin Psychiatry 58:341–347, 1997

Singer HS: Motor stereotypies. Semin Pediatr Neurol 16:77–81, 2009

Teng EJ, Woods DW, Twohig MP, et al: Body-focused repetitive behavior problems: prevalence in a nonreferred population and differences in perceived somatic activity. Behav Modif 26:340–360, 2002

Tolin DF, Franklin ME, Diefenbach GJ, et al: Pediatric trichotillomania: descriptive psychopathology and an open trial of cognitive behavioral therapy. Cogn Behav Ther 36:129–144, 2007

Watson TS, Allen KD: Elimination of thumb-sucking as a treatment for severe trichotillomania. J Am Acad Child Adolesc Psychiatry 32:830–834, 1993

Watson TS, Dittmer KI, Ray KP: Treating trichotillomania in a toddler: variation on effective treatments. Child Fam Behav Ther 22:29–40, 2000

Wilhelm S, Keuthen NJ, Deckersbach T, et al: Self-injurious skin picking: clinical characteristics and comorbidity. J Clin Psychiatry 60:454–459, 1999

Woods DW, Piacentini J, Himle MB, et al: Premonitory Urge for Tics Scale (PUTS): initial psychometric results and examination of the premonitory urge phenomenon in youths with tic disorders. J Dev Behav Pediatr 26:397–403, 2005

Woods DW, Flessner CA, Franklin ME, et al: The Trichotillomania Impact Project (TIP): exploring phenomenology, functional impairment, and treatment utilization. J Clin Psychiatry 67:1877–1888, 2006a

Woods DW, Wetterneck CT, Flessner CA: A controlled evaluation of acceptance and commitment therapy plus habit reversal for trichotillomania. Behav Res Ther 44:639–656, 2006ba

Wright HH, Holmes GR: Trichotillomania (hair pulling) in toddlers. Psychol Rep 92:228–230, 2003

Chapter 6

DERMATOLOGICAL ASSESSMENT OF HAIR PULLING, SKIN PICKING, AND NAIL BITING

Ladan Mostaghimi, M.D.

This chapter offers strategies and methods for distinguishing frequent forms of alopecia, skin eruptions, and nail problems from impulsive hair pulling, skin picking, and nail biting.

CLINICAL APPROACH TO HAIR PULLING

Types of Alopecia

Patients with hair-pulling problems usually seek dermatology help for treatment of alopecia. Once the diagnosis of trichotillomania is made, they may be referred to a psychiatrist for treatment. Many patients are ashamed of hair-pulling behavior and will not admit to it or discuss it, even when they are under psychiatric care for other reasons. Patients who admit to hair pulling do not pose a clinical problem, but if a patient denies hair pulling, other causes of alopecia need to be considered.

Knowledge of the different types of alopecia and their clinical pictures will help in determining the appropriate diagnosis, workup, and treatment.

Alopecia can be characterized as scarring or nonscarring. If the hair follicles are not permanently damaged, the resulting alopecia is *nonscarring*, and once the cause is treated, the hair grows back. In nonscarring alopecia, inspection of the scalp reveals the follicular openings. *Scarring alopecia* occurs when the follicles are permanently damaged and normal hair growth does not resume after the cause of the follicular damage is treated. In this case, the follicular openings are replaced by scar tissue and are not visible. Trichotillomania at its earlier stages is reversible, but once pulling behavior continues for an extended period of time, the repeated stress on hair follicles can result in permanent damage to follicles and scarring alopecia.

Table 6–1 summarizes the different types of alopecia with their respective causes.

Dermatological Assessment of Alopecia

The steps outlined below will assist in the diagnosis of alopecia.

History

A timeline of hair loss and the patient's medical history are important components in the diagnosis of alopecia. A known medical history of systemic diseases such as hyperthyroidism or of taking medications that cause hair loss may suggest a diagnosis of alopecia secondary to systemic problems. The timeline also is important, because some types of alopecia (e.g., alopecia areata) have a more sudden onset than others.

Clinical Examination

The next step is the clinical examination. Does alopecia affect only scalp hair, or are other areas of the body involved (e.g., eyebrows, eyelashes, pubic area)? Trichotillomania can affect not only scalp hair but other areas of the body as well.

In *alopecia areata* (nondiffuse forms), the patches of alopecia are smooth and pale and either round or oval. Around a patch of alopecia are small hairs with thinning proximal shafts (exclamation point hair). Alopecia areata has a polygenic inheritance pattern, and 20%–40% of patients have a family history of alopecia areata (Mounsey and Reed 2009). Hair loss is usually sudden and fast, unlike the gradual hair loss of trichotillomania. Alopecia areata may extend to the entire scalp (alopecia totalis) or entire body (alopecia universalis).

In *trichotillomania*, patches of hair loss often have an irregular shape. The patch contains broken hairs of different lengths. In patients with skin picking in addition to hair pulling, superficial erosions with underlying inflammation and erythema are visible.

The hair pull is a quick clinical test to distinguish trichotillomania from problems arising from the hair follicle. It is done by grasping 40–60 hairs between thumb and index finger and pulling them by applying moderate traction while moving the fingers toward the distal shaft. The test is abnormal if more than 10% of the hair is pulled off (Mounsey and Reed 2009). This test is negative in trichotillomania because there is no real pathology in the hair follicles.

Another type of alopecia, *male or female pattern alopecia*, causes thinning in the vertex and frontotemporal areas of the scalp in men. It is less severe and more diffuse in women. In female pattern alopecia, there is a clear widening of the part in the crown compared with the occipital area of the scalp because hair remains fairly intact in the occipital area. The areas of thinning show miniaturized hair shafts but no broken hairs. Male or female pattern alopecia is androgen dependent and hereditary (Sperling 2009). People with trichotillomania are more likely to seek treatment if they are also affected with male or female pattern alopecia because they will have more difficulty covering bald spots created by trichotillomania.

Examination of alopecia also needs to consider *telogen effluvium*. Telogen effluvium is an acute diffuse hair loss that happens several months (1–6 months) (Hughes 2010) after a physiological or emotional stress, due to early entry of hair follicles into the telogen phase (resting hair). It is usually acute and reversible. Chronic telogen effluvium shows a chronic pattern of hair loss that lasts more than 6 months. Despite excess shedding, follow-up of four patients over a 7-year period in one study did not show a decrease in hair volume (Sinclair 2005). In a normal scalp, 90%–95% of hair follicles are in anagen (growth) phase and the remaining follicles (5%–10%) are in telogen phase. The rate of normal hair loss is approximately 50–100 hairs per day. Clinical examination in telogen effluvium shows diffuse hair loss and no broken hair. Telogen effluvium can occur in newborns and during the postpartum period. It can also occur in the context of severe infections, use of some medications, cancer, thyroid problems, autoimmune problems, end-stage renal and liver diseases, crash dieting, anorexia nervosa, iron deficiency, and protein deficiencies. Medications that most frequently cause telogen effluvium include retinoids, antiepileptic medications (e.g., carbamazepine), beta-blockers, anticoagulants, propylthiouracil, and heavy metals (Sperling 2009).

Telogen effluvium is reversible when the cause is found and treated. However, some cases remain idiopathic. A trichogram (hair pluck and microscopic examination of hairs) will show a mixture of anagen (actively growing) and telogen (resting) hairs. If the percentage of telogen hairs is more than 15%, this is an indicator of abnormal shedding (Sperling 2009). On microscopic examination, telogen hairs have club-shaped ends and anagen hairs have broomstick-shaped and pigmented ends. Anagen effluvium occurs during the use of anticancer medications and is due to impairment of the normal activities (mitotic and metabolic) of hair follicles.

TABLE 6–1.   Classification of causes and types of alopecia

	Scarring (cicatricial)	Nonscarring (noncicatricial)
Diffuse	Burn Congenital atrichia with papules Lipedematous scalp (lipedematous alopecia) Post radiation	Alopecia totalis Alopecia universalis Autoimmune diseases such as systemic lupus erythematosus Telogen effluvium Anagen effluvium Female pattern alopecia Male pattern alopecia Infectious diseases such as syphilis Thyroid disorders (hypo- and hyperthyroidism) Pituitary problems (hyper- and hypopituitarism) Drug induced Iron deficiency Malnutrition (deficiencies in zinc, selenium, iron, biotin, essential fatty acids, protein) Post radiation

TABLE 6–1. Classification of causes and types of alopecia *(continued)*

	Scarring (cicatricial)	Nonscarring (noncicatricial)
Focal	Later stages of trichotillomania	Tinea capitis
	Discoid lupus erythematosus	Alopecia areata
	Lichen planopilaris	Early stages of trichotillomania
	Late stages of traction alopecia	Early stages of traction alopecia
	Alopecia mucinosa	
	Cutaneous T-cell lymphoma and mycosis fungoides	
	Burn	
	Morphea	
	Post radiation	
	Sarcoidosis	
	Tuberculosis	
	Kerion (advance tinea infection and severe host response)	
	Central centrifugal cicatricial alopecia	
	Frontal fibrosing alopecia	
	Acne keloidalis	
	Dissecting cellulitis of the scalp	
	Keratosis pilaris atrophicans	

Infections such as syphilis and HIV can cause hair loss and should be distinguished from trichotillomania. They are usually accompanied by constitutional symptoms (e.g., fever, weight loss) and skin eruption. Individuals at risk for either syphilis or HIV should be tested for both using simple blood tests.

Another possible cause of alopecia is *tinea capitis*. Tinea capitis causes round patches of alopecia associated with redness and scaling. Sometimes the patch may not be red and will resemble seborrheic dermatitis (white to yellowish flaky scales). A Wood lamp examination (a device emitting 365 nanometer–range ultraviolet light) in a dark room may reveal different color fluorescence of the scales based on different infectious agents. Normal skin does not fluoresce with a Wood's lamp. Scraping of scales and KOH testing (potassium hydroxide is used to detect fungi in this test) (Sperling 2009), as well as fungal smear and culture, will reveal the presence of fungi. Treatment will usually reverse the alopecia, except in kerion, in which severe inflammatory reaction to fungus infection leads to scarring alopecia. In "black dot" tinea capitis, the infected broken hairs leave dark stubs visible in the follicular orifice, and this condition needs to be differentiated from trichotillomania.

Traction alopecia is usually due to specific hairstyles that cause repeated plucking of hair in the same area of the scalp. Tight headbands, braids, or ponytails will lead to traction on hair roots and shedding. The clinical picture and pathology resemble those in trichotillomania. Distribution of hair loss and questions concerning the methods used to style hair will help to distinguish this condition from trichotillomania.

Other forms of alopecia (Table 6–1) involve more inflammation than trichotillomania. For example, red papules surround hair follicles in lichen planopilaris and alopecia mucinosa. Erythematous plaques and scarring hair loss are present in cutaneous T-cell lymphomas. In inflammatory alopecia, skin eruptions can be present in other areas of the body, and a complete skin examination will facilitate the diagnosis. Itching is another sign that accompanies many inflammatory types of alopecia and helps to differentiate them from trichotillomania.

Laboratory Investigations

Laboratory tests for alopecia are based on a careful history, review of systems, and physical examination and depend on the suspected diagnosis.

A complete blood count with differential, iron studies, thyroid function tests, kidney function tests, liver function tests, hyperandrogenemia screening in women (total and free testosterone, dehydroepiandrosterone sulfate, and 17α-hydroxyprogesterone), and rapid plasma reagin tests are some of the tests that help with diagnosis of frequent causes of hair loss. KOH testing, as well as a fungal smear and culture of scrapings of the scalp, is done if fungal infection is suspected. Microscopic examination of hair after hair pluck or the hair pull test helps to determine the percentage of anagen versus telogen hairs and shows any abnormalities of the hair shaft.

If the diagnosis is still in doubt, a scalp biopsy is helpful. Usually two 4-mm punch biopsies are performed, one from the area of hair loss and one from the periphery of the lesion (normal scalp for comparison). Histology in trichotillomania shows no significant inflammation. Follicles are of normal size. Disrupted hair follicles together with trichomalacia and pigment casts are other findings in trichotillomania, as shown in Figures 6–1 and 6–2.

CLINICAL APPROACH TO SKIN PICKING

Clinical Characteristics

Skin picking is seen in different clinical situations and can be due to dermatological diseases that cause itching or to impulsive behaviors (neurotic excoriations, acne excoriée) or other psychological problems. A dermatological workup is important to determine the reason for picking.

Many dermatological diseases are accompanied by *itch*. Itch usually leads to scratching that will create erosions, excoriations, and scarring of the skin. A careful clinical examination shows primary lesions (e.g., papules, plaques) if there are any. Some diseases such as dermatitis herpetiformis (a bullous skin disease) cause such severe itching that often the primary skin lesions (vesicles and bullae) are scratched and not easily found.

Neurotic excoriations refers to intentionally produced skin lesions to satisfy a psychological need. Tension is built before scratching/excoriating/picking the skin and is relieved by impulsive picking. Patients may pick at scabs, acne lesions, and other imperfections of their skin, or they may pick normal skin. The lesions are usually located in areas that are reachable and not in areas that are hard to reach. This creates the "butterfly sign" on the back, with a clear area in the shape of butterfly wings. However, this sign is absent in individuals who use other objects besides their fingernails to pick and manipulate their skin (i.e., back scratchers). Patients may use fingernails as well as tweezers, scalpels, or needles to scratch and pick. Based on the method used to scratch, resulting scars may be linear, round, or irregularly shaped.

Sometimes scarring of deep wounds creates *milia*. Milia are small white papules filled with dead skin that is trapped at the base of a hair follicle or sweat gland as a result of scarring and clogging of pores. Primary milia happen without trauma and usually are seen on the face of adults and infants. Secondary milia happen after burns, blistering skin diseases, and dermal injury.

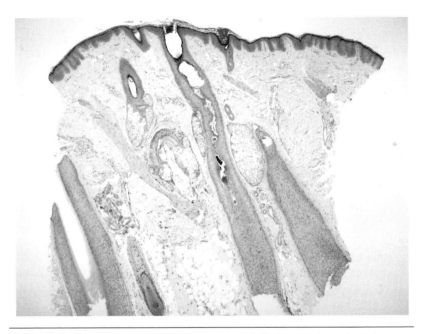

FIGURE 6–1. Spiral pigmented cast in hair follicle in trichomalacia (seen at low power; H & E 4×).

Source. Slide courtesy of Jack Longely, M.D., Professor and Vice Chair of Dermatopathology, University of Wisconsin, Madison.

If there is a secondary gain in picking, the disorder is classified as malingering. If there is no apparent reason for picking, it could be a factitious disorder (to assume the sick role) (Mostaghimi 2010) or an impulse-control disorder.

Some patients deny skin picking and are referred to psychiatry once a dermatology workup has failed to show any primary skin disease. This may cause resentment and anger in patients, and thus building a good therapeutic alliance in this type of clinical situation is important. Referral to a psychocutaneous specialist, if one is available, may improve the outcome. If a psychocutaneous specialist is not available, the psychiatrist needs to work closely with the patient's dermatologist.

Once a therapeutic alliance is built, the psychiatrist should review the clinical workup and continue to be vigilant with clinical symptoms. Some blistering skin diseases such as bullous pemphigoid may start with itching and scratching, followed by blistering later in the course of the disease. In these cases, the initial presentation is urticaria-like red itchy patches that are excoriated without any blisters. Even when the initial dermatology workup is negative, continued clinical vigilance is the rule.

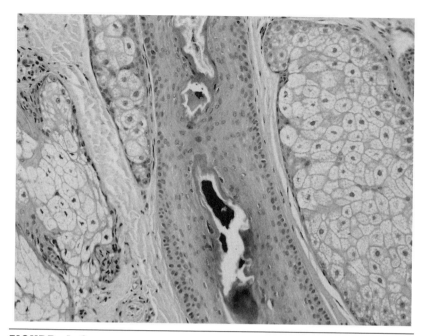

FIGURE 6–2. Spiral pigment cell cast within the follicular lumen in trichomalacia (seen at high power; H & E 20×).

The changes are typical of trichotillomania but could also be seen in other forms of trauma and, rarely, in inflammatory alopecias such as alopecia areata.

Source. Slide courtesy of Jack Longely, M.D., Professor and Vice Chair of Dermatopathology, University of Wisconsin, Madison.

Lesions due to skin picking are more prominent in the areas reachable with the dominant hand and their distribution is asymmetrical, whereas most dermatological diseases have symmetrical distribution. Patients often have long, ragged fingernails with debris and bloodstains under the nails.

Rubbing of skin leads to thickening and accentuation of skin lines (lichenification). Rubbing and consequent lichenification may happen in combination with skin picking, in which case clinical examination will show lichenified plaques in addition to excoriations.

Some patients with skin picking will experience frequent infections and may need topical, oral, or even intravenous antibiotics for bacteremia/septicemia (Odlaug and Grant 2008). I have observed severe joint infections and a case of endocarditis after bacteremia in a patient with severe, chronic skin picking. For these reasons, psychiatrists need to be vigilant and familiar with symptoms of skin infections, including cellulitis. Close collaboration with a dermatologist for skin care in patients with skin picking is the rule.

Psychiatric disorders that can lead to skin picking include impulse-control disorders, anxiety disorders (i.e., obsessive-compulsive disorder), agitated depression, body dysmorphic disorder, delusional disorder (delusion of parasitosis), borderline personality disorder, and developmental disabilities associated with self-injurious behavior. It is important to distinguish dermatology disorders from psychiatric conditions, because even though behavior therapy is important in both conditions for breaking the itch/scratch cycle, the other treatment modalities are very different.

Dermatological Assessment of Skin Picking

Dermatological disorders that have scratching/picking as part of their clinical manifestations include most skin diseases that cause itching. Disorders that are frequently accompanied by scratching and picking include scabies, pediculosis, atopic dermatitis, blistering skin disorders (e.g., bullous pemphigoid, dermatitis herpetiformis), Grover disease, lichen planus, psoriasis, prurigo nodularis, lichen simplex chronicus, and pruritus of different origins, such as uremic pruritus or pruritus accompanying other systemic diseases (e.g., lymphomas, liver failure).

Clinical Examination

Clinical symptoms are used to help distinguish these disorders.

Scabies and *pediculosis* are parasitic disorders that cause severe itching. In patients who take frequent showers, it may be hard to find the culprit agent. Pediculosis (infestation with lice) causes infestation of hairy parts of the body and clothing. Body lice live in clothing and feed on skin. Lice infestation often affects people who live in crowded areas with poor hygiene. Scabies is an infestation with a mite, *Sarcoptes scabiei*, that burrows into the skin and causes severe itching. The mite infestation causes itchy red papules and blisters and linear excoriations in the webs between fingers and toes, and on wrists, extensor elbows, ankles, feet, the waist, nipples, the umbilicus, armpits, buttocks, and genital areas. In some patients, delusions of parasitosis are triggered after an episode of real infestation. Also, some patients may have an irritant dermatitis caused by overtreating the infestation. The eruption and itch/scratch cycle are perpetuated by the treatment itself. This condition needs to be differentiated from the real infestation because treatment is different.

Atopic dermatitis, a pruritic skin disorder that usually starts in infancy and may continue into adulthood, occurs in individuals with a low threshold for different environmental allergens (e.g., dust mites). It may be associated with asthma, allergic rhinitis, food allergies, or other allergies. It is multifactorial in nature, with genetic, immunological, and environmental components. The two main hypotheses for the development of lesions are the immune hypothesis (the problem is due to an imbalance of type 1 and type 2 T helper cells) and the skin barrier function deficiency hypothesis (Krafchik 2010). Patients have severe itching and eczematous eruption with vesicles, crusting, lichenification, and xerosis (dryness) of the skin. Lesions are distributed on cheeks and extensor surfaces of the body in infants and will gradually localize to flexor surfaces (i.e., flexor elbow, posterior knee). Stress plays an important role in triggering flares of atopic dermatitis, and current research shows that psychoneuroimmunological factors are important in the evolution of atopic dermatitis (Arndt et al. 2008). A study in children with atopic dermatitis showed an attenuated hypothalamus-pituitary-adrenal axis response to stress in these children, which may explain the triggering of skin lesions with stress (Buske-Kirschbaum et al. 1997). The blunted response has also been shown in other types of chronic allergic inflammatory reactions (Buske-Kirschbaum et al. 2003). Many children with atopic dermatitis show an increase in picking and skin rubbing when stressed. Picking and rubbing could become a habit, and patients may rub or scratch even without any apparent skin lesions. Family history, the appearance of lesions, and the course of illness help in making the diagnosis.

Blistering skin disorders usually are easily identified by finding bullae on the skin. However, patients with some of these disorders may present with severe itching and excoriations with no apparent primary lesions, and these conditions need to be distinguished from skin picking due to psychological factors.

Bullous pemphigoid is a chronic autoimmune blistering skin disease that is due to production of autoantibodies against hemidesmosomes in the basement membrane (dermo-epidermal junction). It is considered a subepidermal blistering disease, and the diagnosis is made by skin biopsy and immunofluorescence studies of skin (direct immunofluorescence) and serum (indirect immunofluorescence). Bullous pemphigoid primarily affects persons in the fifth to seventh decades of life. The diagnosis is easy when the tense bullae are present, but sometimes the disease starts with a prodromal phase with urticaria-like red patches and itching without any blisters. Histology in this phase usually shows a specific pattern called *eosinophilic spongiosis.* Although not specific to bullous pemphigoid, this pattern can help to differentiate this disease from skin picking that shows epidermal necrosis, focal ulceration, and signs of external trauma to the skin with no inflammation unless a superimposed infection is present.

Dermatitis herpetiformis is a chronic, intensely itchy skin eruption due to gluten sensitivity and associated with gluten-sensitive enteropathy (Miller and Zaman 2009). The clinical course is one of a waxing and waning itchy skin eruption distributed on the extensor surfaces of the extremities (elbows, knees) as well as buttocks and forehead. It may be more generalized and is usually symmetrical. The small blisters are usually ruptured because of severe itching and scratching; other skin lesions include excoriated erythematous papules and urticaria-like plaques. Lesions are polymorphic and may get confused with impulsive skin picking. Clinical course, biopsy with an immunofluorescence study, analysis of serum markers such as immunoglobulin A endomysial antibodies (these could be negative in 10%–37% of cases; Chan 2010), and testing for tissue transglutaminase (not specific to dermatitis herpetiformis; could be positive in other autoimmune diseases; Chan 2010) may help in making the correct diagnosis.

Grover disease (transient acantholytic dermatosis) is a disease that frequently affects middle-aged white men but may affect females and other ethnic groups. The etiology is unknown, and although the disease is generally considered benign with a short course, it may be chronic in some cases. Grover disease is usually limited to the chest and upper back but may be generalized or unilateral in some cases. It is accompanied by different degrees of itching. Primary lesions, including papules, pustules, or vesicles, are present. The presence of primary lesions and a skin biopsy will help to differentiate it from skin picking.

Lichen planus is a chronic inflammatory autoimmune disease of the skin and mouth. On the skin, lichen planus manifests with aggregation of very itchy flat-top papules, some of which have a lacy white surface (Wickham striae). It usually affects flexor wrists and the inner side of ankles, but it may be seen anywhere on the body. Primary lesions are easy to find, and the diagnosis can be confirmed by skin biopsy and histology if there is any doubt. In the mouth, lichen planus causes painful erosions and white lacy patches inside the cheeks but can affect other areas of the mouth as well (gums, lips, tongue).

Psoriasis is a chronic inflammatory papulosquamous skin disease. It has various clinical presentations, including red, well-defined patches and plaques covered with silvery scales, small white scaly papules, and hyperkeratotic dry skin with cracks and fissures (on palmoplantar areas of skin). It can affect the scalp and nails. The usual distribution is symmetrical on extensor surfaces, except in inverse psoriasis. The lesions can cause intense itching. Emotional stress makes the itching worse. Some patients may pick at the scales, and this will aggravate the lesions as a result of koebnerization. The Koebner phenomenon occurs when new plaques of psoriasis appear on an injured area of skin. Treating the psoriasis and working on breaking the itch/scratch cycle with behavior therapy will help improve the skin. Many patients with psoriasis will benefit from psychological counseling.

Prurigo nodularis, also called *chronic circumscribed nodular lichenification* and *Picker's nodules* (Lotti et al. 2008), is a chronic dermatological disease with papules and nodules that are extremely itchy and often have excoriated, warty, pigmented surfaces. The lesions are usually distributed on the extensor surface of limbs and occasionally on the face and trunk. Breaking the itch/scratch cycle is an important part of the treatment of prurigo nodularis, and psychiatrists should not be surprised if a patient with this type of skin eruption is referred by his or her dermatologist to psychiatry for treatment.

Lichen simplex chronicus is caused by excessive rubbing and scratching, leading to lichenification of the skin (Mostaghimi 2010). Patients have plaques of thickened skin in the occipital scalp, neck, extensor forearms, ankles, and genital areas. Lichen simplex chronicus, like prurigo nodularis, has itch as its main symptom and is worsened by emotional stress.

Psychological intervention and psychotropic medications are helpful for some patients with prurigo nodularis or lichen simplex chronicus, and dermatologists often refer patients with intractable itching to psychocutaneous specialists or psychiatrists for treatment.

Pruritus, or itching of the skin, can be due to general medical problems (e.g., thyroid, parathyroid, liver, or kidney problems; lymphomas; medication side effects; iron deficiency). It will usually lead to scratching and may be confused with impulsive skin picking.

Laboratory Investigations

Workup of itching and skin picking is based on clinical symptoms and may include the following:

- Scrapping and microscopic examination of the lesions for scabies
- Wood lamp examination for fungal infections
- Patch testing for allergies
- Complete blood count with differential (watch for hypereosinophilic syndromes and lymphomas)
- Iron studies
- Stool check for parasites
- Gastrointestinal testing to look for malabsorption and gluten sensitivity
- Thyroid, parathyroid, liver, and kidney functions and fasting blood sugar
- Rapid plasma reagin and HIV testing (if indicated)
- Skin biopsy together with direct and indirect immunofluorescence (if bullous dermatosis is suspected)
- Computed tomography scan and chest X ray (if lymphoma is suspected)

CLINICAL APPROACH TO NAIL BITING

Clinical Characteristics

Nail biting is a frequent compulsive behavior that causes damage to nails. It is more frequent in children and adolescents. Using the search term "nail biting" in Google's image search engine locates clinical pictures of characteristic changes in affected nails. Many people with skin picking may also have nail biting. The same patient may have nail biting, skin picking, and hair pulling in different periods of his or her life. It is not uncommon that one behavior replaces another.

The nail plate is produced by the nail matrix. It grows from the proximal nail fold and progresses distally; it adheres to the nail bed. Fingernails grow 3 mm per month and toenails grow 1 mm per month (Tosti and Piraccini 2009). Nail biting affects the nail plate and proximal nail fold. Trauma to the nail matrix will produce nail plate abnormalities. There is destruction of the distal part of the nail plate due to biting. Nails are short and ragged and show subungual hemorrhage. Periungual inflammation, erythema, erosions, and crusting may be present. Chronic nail biting causes stress on teeth and leads to cracking, chipping, and wearing down of the front teeth. In people with tics involving rubbing or touching of the proximal nail fold, dystrophy may be present and should be differentiated from matrix tumors causing nail dystrophy.

Dermatological Assessment of Nail Problems

Nails are affected in different skin diseases (e.g., psoriasis, alopecia areata, lichen planus, eczema) as well as systemic diseases (e.g., iron deficiency, connective tissue disorders, peripheral neuropathies, HIV infection, cardiovascular diseases, endocrine diseases, pulmonary diseases). Nail abnormalities can be induced by infectious agents (e.g., tinea, *Candida*, *Pseudomonas*, viral warts, herpes), nail tumors (e.g., melanoma, squamous cell carcinoma), or drugs (e.g., chemotherapy agents, cyclines, nonsteroidal anti-inflammatory drugs, psoralens, zidovudine and other anti-HIV medications, antimalarials, gold, retinoids, methotrexate, beta-blockers) (Tosti and Piraccini 2009) or may be congenital.

Inflammation of the nail fold, called *paronychia*, can be acute or chronic. Occasionally, nail-biting habits, especially if they damage the cuticles, lead to paronychia and superimposed infections.

Different problems in nails produce different clinical pictures. If patients deny nail biting, other problems that cause nail symptoms need to be ruled out. A good history and physical examination help to differentiate nail biting from other dermatological or systemic problems.

When gathering the patient's history, the clinician should carefully note the timeline of the problem (acute vs. chronic) and medication history, as well as the presence of systemic symptoms.

Clinical Picture

Nail biting usually affects fingernails because of their easy accessibility; all or some of the fingernails may be affected. A complete skin examination may show psoriasis plaques, eczema lesions, lichen planus, or signs of other dermatological diseases elsewhere on the body. Systemic and congenital problems affect multiple nails, including toenails, and are usually symmetrical. Congenital problems may also be accompanied by hair and teeth problems. Tumors often affect a single nail.

Change in nail color is seen in cases of drug reactions, infections, or tumors. Nail biting per se does not cause thickening or change of color in nails unless there is a superimposed infection.

Bad habits other than nail biting, such as repeated and rigorous hand washing in patients with obsessive-compulsive disorder, may cause damage and brittleness of the nails. Damage to nails may be seen in eating disorders as a result of nutritional deficiencies.

In summary, a good history and physical examination will lead to an appropriate diagnosis, workup, and treatment.

Laboratory Investigations

Laboratory tests are based on clinical examination and consist of the following:

- Blood check for systemic diseases if any suspicion
- Fungal smear and culture as well as microbial culture of affected nails
- Biopsy of the affected nail by a dermatologist in case of suspicion of tumors

CONCLUSION

Psychiatrists who are treating patients with alopecia, skin eruption, or nail problems need to work closely with a dermatologist. Continued vigilance is the rule, because even patients with no primary dermatology disorder may have superimposed infections that need appropriate treatment.

Specific clinical scenarios in which close collaboration between dermatologist and psychiatrist is needed include the following:

- Patients requesting cosmetic treatments (e.g., laser, peeling) for scars created by skin picking need to know that as long as skin picking continues, treatment of scars will not be of any help and will only create excessive financial hardship for them.
- Patients with skin picking who require surgical procedures unrelated to the repetitive behavior are at risk for infections at the surgical site due to picking. Appropriate support and therapy are needed until the surgical wound heals.

REFERENCES

Arndt J, Smith N, Tausk F: Stress and atopic dermatitis. Curr Allergy Asthma Rep 8:312–317, 2008

Buske-Kirschbaum A, Jobst S, Wustmans A, et al: Attenuated free cortisol response to psychosocial stress in children with atopic dermatitis. Psychosom Med 59:419–426, 1997

Buske-Kirschbaum A, von Auer K, Krieger S, et al: Blunted cortisol responses to psychosocial stress in asthmatic children: a general feature of atopic disease? Psychosom Med 65:806–810, 2003

Chan L: Bullous pemphigoid, in eMedicine from WebMD, 2010. Available at: http://emedicine.medscape.com/article/1062391-overview. Accessed December 12, 2010.

Hughes ECW: Telogen effluvium, in eMedicine from WebMD, 2010. Available at: http://emedicine.medscape.com/article/1071566-overview. Accessed December 12, 2010.

Krafchik BR: Atopic dermatitis, in eMedicine from WebMD, 2010. Available at: http://emedicine.medscape.com/article/1049085-overview. Accessed December 12, 2010.

Lotti T, Buggiani G, Prignano F: Prurigo nodularis and lichen simplex chronicus. Dermatol Ther 21:42–46, 2008

Miller JL, Zaman SA: Dermatitis herpetiformis, in eMedicine from WebMD, 2009. Available at: http://emedicine.medscape.com/article/1062640-overview. Accessed January 24, 2010.

Mostaghimi L: Psychocutaneous medicine, in Conn's Current Therapy, 10th Edition. Edited by Bope ET, Rakel RE, Kellerman RD. Philadelphia, PA, Saunders Elsevier, 2010, pp 793–798

Mounsey AL, Reed SW: Diagnosing and treating hair loss. Am Fam Physician 80:356–362, 2009

Odlaug BL, Grant JE: Clinical characteristics and medical complications of pathologic skin picking. Gen Hosp Psychiatry 30:61–66, 2008

Sinclair R: Chronic telogen effluvium: a study of 5 patients over 7 years. J Am Acad Dermatol 52:12–16, 2005

Sperling LC: Alopecia, in Dermatology, 2nd Edition. Edited by Bolognia JL, Jorizzo JL, Rapini RP. Philadelphia, PA, Elsevier, 2009

Tosti A, Piraccini BM: Nail disorders, in Dermatology, 2nd Edition. Edited by Bolognia JL, Jorizzo JL, Rapini RP. Philadelphia, PA, Elsevier, 2009, pp 1061–1078

Chapter 7

DIAGNOSIS AND EVALUATION

Trichotillomania, Skin Picking, and
Other Stereotypic Behaviors in Children

Martin E. Franklin, Ph.D.
Diana Antinoro, Psy.D.
Kristin Benavides, B.A.

Our task in the current chapter is to provide an examination of the diagnosis and assessment of trichotillomania, pathological skin picking (PSP), and related problems in children and adolescents. The extant literature on these conditions in youth has burgeoned since 2000, but significant holes remain in our knowledge base with respect to epidemiology, psychopathology, underlying neurobiology, and treatment response. Assessment tools for the core symptoms of trichotillomania in youth have been developed recently and their psychometric properties examined (Flessner et al. 2007; Tolin et al. 2008), but comparable progress has not been made as yet for pediatric skin picking and related problems. Regardless of the state of current scientific knowledge, many families present clinically for assistance for their child who engages in such behaviors, and thus we simply do not have the luxury of waiting for the empirical literature to become more fully informative.

Before reviewing specific assessment strategies and tools, we describe briefly what we know about the course of these disorders over development; discuss specific similarities and differences in presentation between children, adolescents, and adults; and present information about what is known about core psychopathology, comorbidity patterns, and association with functional impairment. This information sets the context for deciding what instruments to use and what areas to survey in gathering the data needed to fully inform the intervention strategies. Regardless of which treatment option is chosen—cognitive-behavioral therapy, pharmacotherapy, both, or other alternatives with fewer empirical data attesting to efficacy—a proper and thorough assessment sets the stage for intervention and informs the clinician about whether treatment is working and, if not, what alternatives should be considered and why.

The term *assessment* involves the integration of information from multiple sources to provide a cohesive understanding of the presenting concern in a context. There are multiple reasons to complete a comprehensive assessment of psychological disorders of all kinds, including trichotillomania and related conditions. Most often, clinical practice relies on accurate assessments to obtain initial diagnoses, to gather information for treatment planning, and to evaluate change in symptom severity. Such assessments typically include presenting symptoms, diagnostic severity, functional impairment, differential diagnosis, comorbidity, and global assessment of functioning. This information assists accurate diagnosis according to the multiaxial structure of DSM-IV-TR (American Psychiatric Association 2000). In this chapter, specific techniques and measures are presented related to the assessment of trichotillomania, skin picking, and other related conditions. The state of the literature is such that the psychometric properties of many, if not most, of the scales in use clinically have not been thoroughly evaluated, which raises some questions as to reliability and validity. Scales that do have such data are clearly identified in the text.

DEVELOPMENTAL COURSE: PHENOMENOLOGY, COMORBIDITY, AND IMPAIRMENT

Trichotillomania has been defined as the recurrent pulling out of one's hair, resulting in hair loss, with an increasing sense of tension before pulling, followed by a feeling of gratification or relief after the pulling episode (American Psychiatric Association 2000). Not all who experience pulling-related hair loss report both tension and relief (e.g., Christenson et al. 1991), and this may especially be the case with children (Hanna 1997; King et al. 1995; Reeve et al. 1992; Wright and Holmes 2003). Hair manipulation in the form of hair twirling, stroking, and pulling appears to be very common in many children and is sometimes associated with habits such as thumb sucking and nail biting (e.g., Byrd et al. 2002). Early-onset (i.e., in toddlers) hair pulling is thought of by some as a benign habit with a shorter course as opposed to trichotillomania, which usually has a later onset, yet research has not empirically confirmed the differences, either in function or in prognosis, between early- and later-onset pulling.

The field lacks definitive, longitudinal assessment studies to identify changes in trichotillomania phenomenology, severity, and comorbidity patterns over the course of development, which significantly hampers our ability to make predictions about changes in course over time. In the absence of longitudinal data, comparisons of cross-sectional data in adults and children suggest developmental differences in the ability to identify affective cues that precede pulling, as well as differences in symptom severity and associated comorbid conditions over the course of development (e.g., Franklin and Tolin 2007). For example, comorbid mood disorders appear to be much more common in adults with trichotillomania than in younger patients, whereas attentional problems such as attention-deficit/hyperactivity disorder (ADHD) appear to be quite common in younger samples and to occur at higher rates than would be expected given their population base rates (e.g., Franklin et al. 2008; Tolin et al. 2007). These studies also suggest that functional impairment appears to grow more pronounced over time from pediatric to adult samples, although this finding is complicated by the fact that comorbidity patterns are also changing and the separate effects of trichotillomania versus the comorbid condition on functioning are difficult to disentangle. In our experience, we have also found that younger children who may not be especially attentive to social context often report less distress and impairment than do adolescents, for whom the social milieu has taken on considerable importance for developmental reasons. There is almost no literature for guidance on these same patterns in skin picking and related conditions, but from our clinical work we have witnessed similar developmental changes in symptom severity, comorbidity patterns, and functional impairment. Assessment strategies, therefore, must be considered accordingly.

THE ASSESSMENT PROCESS

What Is the Role of Assessment in Treatment?

The importance of an adequate assessment in treatment planning is evident across all theoretical approaches to therapy. Simply, it is essential to know the patient's basic information in order to treat the presenting concern. Furthermore, empirically based treatments rely heavily on these data to identify the optimal or most effective treatment according to current research and clinical practice recommendations. Specifically, cognitive-behavioral interventions, which are recommended by experts for trichotillomania and related disorders (Flessner et al. 2010), use these assessment data to identify appropriate interventions and tailor the treatment to the particular patient and symptoms.

The theoretical underpinnings of cognitive-behavioral treatments for trichotillomania and related disorders are based on the functional relationships between the symptoms and the patient's needs. This function-based approach depends greatly on behavioral theory and more specifically on the behavioral concepts of reinforcement. *Reinforcement*, or *operant conditioning*, may be defined as environmental events or consequences that occur in response to a behavior that will increase the likelihood that the behavior will occur again in the future (Cooper et al. 1990). For instance, when a child throws a tantrum for a candy bar and the parent gives the child the candy bar to stop the crying, the child will be more likely to cry the next time he or she desires something (especially candy bars). Reinforcement exists in two forms: positive and negative reinforcement. Positive reinforcement consists of the addition of a stimulus to the environment (a candy bar) that will increase the likelihood of the behavior, whereas negative reinforcement includes the removal of a stimulus from the environment (annoying buzzing from the alarm clock) that will increase the likelihood of the behavior. Both forms include an increase or maintenance of the behavior.

The presence of positive and negative reinforcement is found with trichotillomania and related disorders. Therefore, assessments must include specific and detailed inquiries about the connections between the symptoms and their antecedents and consequences. For instance, anxiety treatment often targets avoidance and escape (negative reinforcement or relief) from the feared object. With this treatment framework, it is assumed that the avoidance maintains the anxiety by providing relief (removal of anxiety or negative reinforcement). Hence, exposure to feared stimuli (not avoidance) will then function as a mechanism to decrease anxiety through habituation.

Additionally, the patient may access positive reinforcement (assistance or attention from friends) that also maintains the anxiety response. Therefore, access to attention and assistance should be sought in alternative manners. These interventions seek to eliminate the function of anxiety behaviors for the patient. Thus, the functional relationship provides the basis for intervention and treatment and is vital to the assessment process. It is optimal for the clinician, when engaging in the assessment, to integrate the incoming information with a potential treatment plan. Utilizing these functional connections will direct the course of the assessment and identify areas in need of further exploration.

Who Should Conduct, and Who Should Be Involved in, the Assessment Process?

Often measures and assessment materials identify the level of education required for the administrator. If this information is not specified by the test creators, it can be assumed that a qualified person would have a master's degree or doctorate in the applied area. Additionally, many structured interviews also recommend specific training in order to provide standardized administration. Overall, psychological education and training are essential to incorporate the plethora of information that often requires differentiating between diagnoses and taking into account many other patient variables, including culture, religion, socioeconomic status, and many other characteristics. This clinical judgment serves to buffer some of the error in our often imperfect measurement instruments.

The age of the child will often dictate whether parents are invited to participate in the entire evaluation meeting with the clinician, with the suggestion that the younger the child, the more important it is to have parents in the room for the entire interview. Within that same context, age and other developmental factors (e.g., shyness, previous experience with interacting with adults) may determine whether questions are directed to the child or to the parent; it is important if both are in the room that the clinician explain that the goal of the meeting is to gather as much information about the pulling as possible and incorporate everyone's perspective rather than to arrive at "the truth." This preemptive strike and subsequent reminders of the overarching purpose of the assessment might minimize the likelihood of conflict when the child and the parent disagree over the details of pulling and over its impact on the child. With adolescents, it is usually preferable to interview the adolescent alone but to invite parents in later to provide a synopsis of the assessment in a way that is respectful of the adolescent's concerns about privacy as well as the parent's needs to understand the clinical recommendations to follow.

How Should Families Be Oriented to the Assessment Process?

The most relevant context for any child who presents to the clinic for treatment is the family context, and it is important to evaluate this context in addition to inquiring about the specific details of the child's repetitive behavior for which the family is seeking help. Before the clinician engages in detailed assessment of a specific disorder, it is helpful to provide psychoeducation about the illness or disorder. This serves to destigmatize the disorder for the patient and the family, allowing them to speak more freely about their experience in an accepting environment. Typically, we provide a range of examples of common symptom presentations that span the gamut of possible symptoms. When discussed in a neutral and matter-of-fact manner, this information allows the patient to feel understood, not judged, and accepted. Ideally, this information also provides a framework within which the patient may understand the assessment questions that follow. It is also strongly recommended that the psychoeducational material presented be supported by the empirical literature to the extent possible, which requires that the clinician conducting this initial meeting be familiar with studies that have examined the clinical presentation and treatment of the problem of relevance. For disorders in which this literature is weak (e.g., skin picking in children), a case should be made about its functional similarity to disorders about which there is more known (e.g., trichotillomania, skin picking in adults), which will allow families to interpolate from studies of similar conditions to their specific problem of focus.

The psychoeducation provided in the context of assessment also serves as a preliminary introduction to the treatment process, providing an opportunity for the patients to assess their goodness of fit with the theoretical concepts that underlie the treatment offered. Sometimes, describing the conceptualization may serve as the initial shift in how the person understands and reacts to current symptoms. This alone may cause change for the patient. For example, there are many times when the presentation of information about post-pulling or post-picking behaviors that other patients have reported (e.g., chewing on roots or eating scabs) will prompt a child to say, "I had no idea that other people did that too!" which then opens the door toward improved rapport, increased knowledge about the condition itself, and decreased defensiveness when discussing its most intimate and critical details. It is especially important, then, that the clinician adopt and retain this open and accepting stance, because responses such as "We see that a lot in the kids we treat who have trichotillomania" or "Actually, most people who pull do report some positive feelings immediately after doing so" serve to provide a context for provision of the most accurate information, which in turn will be most informative when it comes to designing and implementing the treatment.

Which Measures Should Be Included to Make the Diagnosis?

There are many approaches to the assessment of psychological disorders, including the use of self-report forms, interviews, and behavioral observation exercises. Depending on the age of the patient and the needed information, an assessment may include all, some, or only one of these. A comprehensive assessment typically includes two formats, often self-reports and interviews. The combination of these formats provides confirmation of the gathered information and an alternate way to access information.

It is optimal to choose a variety of report formats to obtain confirmation for the collected material. Often, clinicians combine self-report and clinician-administered measures so they may integrate the patient's perspective, facts, and clinical judgment. Determining which measures to use should take time constraints and cost constraints into consideration.

Trichotillomania Diagnostic Interview

The Trichotillomania Diagnostic Interview (TDI; Rothbaum and Ninan 1994) is often used as an intake measure to establish a diagnosis of DSM-IV (American Psychiatric Association 1994) trichotillomania. The TDI is a sem-istructured interview that entails a three-point clinician rating of each DSM-IV (or DSM-IV-TR) criterion for trichotillomania. It affords an advance over unstructured clinical interview techniques in that it ensures each criterion is investigated and allows for ratings to indicate threshold, subthreshold, and absent symptomatology. The TDI is easy and quick to administer. It requires minimal training or practice besides the typical experiences with diagnosis and psychopathology.

The TDI contains six items; for a diagnosis to be made, the patient must report that the onset of hair-pulling behaviors was 6 months prior to the assessment and that there is significant distress associated with the pulling. As in all DSM-IV-TR diagnoses, individuals with trichotillomania cannot have their disturbance better accounted for by another mental disorder or general medical condition. The less developmentally sensitive criteria for trichotillomania include increasing tension prior to pulling; and pleasure, gratification, or relief when pulling. Although these criteria are needed for a diagnosis of trichotillomania according to DSM-IV-TR, they do not provide a good indicator of clinical interference or need for treatment, especially among younger patients. Therefore, in clinical practice these items are often not necessary to warrant treatment.

Measures of Disorder-Specific Symptoms

A comprehensive functional assessment of hair-pulling behaviors often leads clinicians to identify boredom and stress or emotion as reliable triggers for pulling episodes. Corresponding consequences include relieving stress and obtaining some types of pleasure (e.g., playing with the hair, mild enjoyment in finding the hair). Even though these appear to be the most common functions identified, there may be other functional relationships for different patients. In addition to ensuring an appropriate diagnosis, it is essential to investigate these and other functions in the assessment process.

Measures for diagnosis and symptom severity often include amount of hair pulled, time spent pulling, frequency of interference, distress level, extent of hair thinning/bald areas, activity limitations, and various other components. This wealth of information provides the clinician with insight into how much the trichotillomania is present in the patient's daily life and how much difficulty it is causing. The measures that follow are specific to trichotillomania, yet there is an additional section toward the end of this chapter on measures recommended to augment this trichotillomania-specific information.

Comparable measures have yet to be developed for children with skin picking and related problems, so the most reasonable clinical strategy to employ in the absence of such instruments is to adapt those already developed for trichotillomania or to make use of instruments developed for adults (e.g., the Massachusetts General Hospital Skin Picking Scale; Keuthen et al. 2001).

Clinician-Administered Measures

National Institute of Mental Health Trichotillomania Questionnaire. Derived from the Yale-Brown Obsessive Compulsive Scale (Goodman et al. 1989a, 1989b), the National Institute of Mental Health (NIMH) Trichotillomania Questionnaire (Swedo et al. 1989) is a semistructured clinical interview consisting of two clinician-rated scales: the NIMH Trichotillomania Severity Scale (NIMH-TSS) and the NIMH Trichotillomania Impairment Scale (NIMH-TIS). The NIMH-TSS consists of five questions related to the following aspects of trichotillomania: average time spent pulling, time spent pulling on the previous day, resistance to urges, resulting distress, and daily interference. NIMH-TSS scores range from 0 to 25. This section of the NIMH-TSS is easily administered in 10–20 minutes. Yet two components often need clarification: distress and interference. In clinical and research practice, it is ideal to provide examples of distress and interference (e.g., anger after pulling, consuming extra time for grooming, avoiding pools) to help separate these two domains. The NIMH-TIS is an impairment scale with scores ranging from 0 to 10. Minimal, mild, and moderate/severe impairment ratings are dependent upon the extent of distress experienced due to trichotillomania, the extent of hair loss, and interference in daily activities. Higher scores on both of the NIMH scales indicate greater severity/impairment.

Psychometric data for the NIMH Trichotillomania Questionnaire are limited, but good interrater reliability was found in one study (Swedo et al. 1989). The NIMH-TSS has been shown to be sensitive to changes in symptom severity and impairment following treatment (Lerner et al. 1998; Rothbaum 1992; Swedo et al. 1989). In a recently completed randomized, controlled trial completed by our group at the University of Pennsylvania, test-retest reliability on all subjects completing intake and baseline ($n=24$) was acceptable (0.70), even with different raters and interviews. The interrater agreement for 50% of that sample between independent evaluator–rated NIMH-TSS total score at baseline and an independent rater was good (0.88).

Photograph measurement.   Another potentially useful objective measure of trichotillomania severity and change following treatment is the use of photographs. Photos are taken of the patient's primary pulling sites, providing a concrete assessment of treatment success (not pulling). It is often best to have photographs taken of the patient's bald areas before and after treatment to assess for these concrete changes. Additionally, the patient may use this photographic record to monitor maintenance and predict relapse.

These photo procedures have been used in previous adult and pediatric trichotillomania studies (e.g., Diefenbach et al. 2005; Rapp et al. 1998; Vitulano et al. 1992). In a recent trial at Penn, good interrater reliability ($r=0.87$) was noted when second ratings were made from photographs of alopecia areas (Tolin et al. 2002). Photographs may also be assessed using a Likert scale to provide for greater precision. In our studies, a seven-point Likert scale ranging from no evidence of alopecia (score of 1) to complete denudement of the area (score of 7) has been implemented. Understandably, patients and possibly even parents may be reticent to permit such a photograph to be taken, and it is up to the clinician to exercise judgment in determining whether the data would be especially helpful in informing treatment.

Self-Report Measures

Milwaukee Inventory for Styles of Trichotillomania—Child Version.   The Milwaukee Inventory for Styles of Trichotillomania—Child Version (MIST-C; Flessner et al. 2007, 2008) is a 25-question measure assessing the style of pulling. A nine-point Likert scale is used to help patients identify their common pattern of pulling, which is characterized as either automatic or focused. Questions on the MIST-C include information about the patient's level of urge awareness, level of active pulling behaviors, and use of implements to pull. The purpose of the measure is to help determine the overall level of pulling awareness. Clinically, many have suggested that automatic pulling is likely more amenable to reduction via standard behavioral methods incorporated into habit-reversal training protocols (see, e.g., Franklin and Tolin 2007), whereas focused pulling may require more clinical attention to the affective cues that often drive this form of pulling. Because the MIST-C surveys this information, it is strongly recommended that clinicians make use of this brief instrument as a routine part of initial and repeated assessment during treatment.

Premonitory Urge for Tics Scale.   The Premonitory Urge for Tics Scale, or PUTS (Woods 2005), is a nine-item self-report questionnaire designed to assess for the presence of premonitory sensory urges common in persons with chronic tic disorders, but can be adapted clinically for use with trichotillomania and related conditions to assess various aspects of urges. Higher scores represent greater levels of premonitory urges. A study of youth with chronic tic disorders indicated that the PUTS was internally consistent ($\alpha = 0.81$) and temporally stable at 2 weeks ($r=0.86$, $P<0.01$), although the data also suggested that very young children (age 9 or younger) were unable to respond reliably to questions about the nature of their urges to engage in tics.

Because urges also appear to be a common and important phenomenon for individuals with trichotillomania, adapting the PUTS for use in assessing urge presence and intensity is strongly recommended. For example, an item on the PUTS reads, "Right before I do a tic, I feel 'wound up' or tense inside." Adapting this measure simply entails interchanging tics for trichotillomania, such as "Right before I pull a hair, I feel 'wound up' or tense inside."

Measures of Functional Impairment

Developed primarily for the research context, the instruments described below nevertheless may have a useful clinical function, which is to quantify the broader effects of trichotillomania on the child or adolescent's day-to-day functioning. Although research has identified a relatively strong relationship between pulling severity and functional impairment (Franklin et al. 2008; Woods et al. 2006), there are individual cases in which even mild symptoms are associated with very severe impairment and other cases in which patients with very high rates of pulling and intense pulling urges continue to function without substantial difficulty. An instrument to document this often complex relationship is helpful in determining where the focus should be in treatment.

Social Adjustment Scale—Self-Report.   The SAS-SR (Weissman et al. 1978) is a self-report measure assessing social adjustment across four major role areas (school behavior, spare time, peer relations, and family behavior). Youngsters rate 21 items on a five-point scale, with higher scores reflecting greater impairment. Both a total adjustment score and separate role area scores are computed. The SAS-SR possesses acceptable psychometrics.

Children's Global Assessment Scale.   The Children's Global Assessment Scale (CGAS; Shaffer et al. 1983) provides a measure of global impairment and functioning over the previous month. The scale ranges from 1 (lowest functioning) to 100 (highest functioning). Green (1994) provided evidence for the psychometric soundness of the CGAS and suggested that ratings obtained in clinical contexts may reflect evaluations of functional competence rather than symptom severity.

Which Measures Should Be Included to Assess Comorbidity?

A semistructured clinical interview is unlikely to be feasible in the clinical context, although there are some instruments, such as the Mini International Neuropsychiatric Interview—Kid (MINI-KID; Sheehan et al. 2010) and the Anxiety Disorders Interview Schedule for Children (ADIS-C; Silverman and Albano 1996) that provide a broad diagnostic survey of the more common comorbid conditions. In the absence of a formal survey of comorbid conditions, however, it is wise to include parent- and self-report instruments to assist in determining whether trichotillomania is primary and whether and how comorbid symptoms should be addressed in the context of treatment planning.

Multidimensional Anxiety Scale for Children

The Multidimensional Anxiety Scale for Children (MASC; March et al. 1997) is a self-report questionnaire for children and adolescents that assesses four broad anxiety domains: physical symptoms, social anxiety, harm avoidance, and separation/panic. It has 39 items, which are scored from 0 (statement never true for you) to 3 (statement often true for you). The MASC shows acceptable internal consistency (0.60–0.85), test-retest reliability (0.77–0.79), and validity (March et al. 1997). The measure is included in light of previous research suggesting a possible relationship between trichotillomania and anxiety (Franklin et al. 2008; Lewin et al. 2009), although the presence of an anxiety disorder was not found to negatively affect the efficacy of trichotillomania-specific behavioral treatment in youth (Franklin and Rae 2010).

Children's Depression Inventory

Depressive symptoms can be evaluated using the Children's Depression Inventory (CDI; Kovacs 1985). The CDI is a self-report scale that inventories cognitive, affective, behavioral, and interpersonal symptoms of depression and has demonstrated adequate psychometric properties (Kovacs 1985). The measure may be especially important to include in light of previous research in youth suggesting a strong, positive correlation between trichotillomania and depressive symptoms (Lewin et al. 2009) and in light of the expectation that significant depressive symptoms and mood disorder diagnoses are the norm in adults with trichotillomania. The presence of significant depressive symptoms must be factored in when clinical recommendations are presented to the family; the mood disorder may well become the primary treatment target in some cases, with trichotillomania treatment commencing after those symptoms have been addressed.

Conners' Parent Rating Scales—Revised.   Parental ratings of their child's internalizing and externalizing symptoms can be surveyed using the Conners' Parent Rating Scale—Revised (CPRS-R; Conners et al. 1998), a reliable and valid instrument utilized in many previous research studies of pediatric psychopathology and its treatment. The CPRS-R yields scores on factors covering both externalizing and internalizing domains; it provides a broad assessment that can then be followed up on clinically. From the standpoint of treatment, comorbid ADHD symptoms are particularly important to identify because such symptoms have previously been associated with attenuated outcomes in studies of obsessive-compulsive disorder and Tourette syndrome in adults and in youth (Deckersbach et al. 2006; Storch et al. 2009).

What Else Do You Need to Know?

An assessment of a child or adolescent with trichotillomania or a related condition is not complete without evaluating the quality of his or her interpersonal relationships both within and outside the family, because treatments that require effort and may produce some distress in the patient (e.g., behavioral approaches) will be enhanced by garnering as much social support as possible from trusted others. Who in the child's life already knows about the problem? What has been their response? Does this response help the child or does it produce more stress, which then further fuels the pulling cycle? Friendships in older children and in adolescents are often their greatest source of support, so it is important to know whether the child has the kind of relationships or relationship development skills that will facilitate this kind of assistance from others. What are his or her academic, athletic, and home activities and responsibilities, and how do these interplay with symptoms? Also, how motivated is the child to engage in treatment, to use treatment techniques that can be cumbersome and difficult to get used to at first, and to tolerate the discomfort or distress that will likely follow if he or she uses certain techniques properly (e.g., competing responses), at least at first? A motivated parent but an unmotivated child is a clinical conundrum, and in our view, if the child's motivation cannot be enhanced, then certain forms of treatment (e.g., pharmacotherapy) may well be more suitable than others (e.g., behavior therapy) that require considerable time, effort, and energy on the child's part.

It is also important to determine how the child likes to think and what his or her interests are, so that treatment metaphors so often employed in psychosocial treatments can be tailored to those interests in order to make the possibly otherwise tedious task of improving awareness of urges, identifying the exact sequence of behaviors that precede the behavior, and examining its consequences at least somewhat less aversive. Kendall's principles of "flexibility within fidelity" certainly apply to the treatment process (Kendall et al. 2008) but also apply to assessment in that the specifics of the assessment protocol can be conveyed more effectively to the child if they are couched in developmentally sensitive language that the child or adolescent finds engaging and interesting rather than dry and intrusive.

BRINGING IT ALL TOGETHER: USING ASSESSMENT DATA TO INFORM CLINICAL DECISION MAKING

A clinician who has spent the time necessary to gather the data described here will be in the best position to make clinical recommendations to the family. Information about trichotillomania diagnosis, symptom severity, functional impairment, and comorbid symptoms and diagnoses can now be taken into account along with family environment and stressors and the child's developmental level, interests, and motivation, allowing the clinician to make suggestions as to which way to proceed clinically. A complex decision tree unfolds based on these data, and the rationale for making one recommendation over another should be fully discussed. Patients whose symptoms of trichotillomania or related conditions are primary, who appear to be highly motivated and willing to engage in therapy, and who are capable of adhering to a weekly treatment regimen for 8–12 weeks might be best served by pursuing behavior therapy (e.g., Bloch et al. 2007), as the meta-analytic data would suggest for trichotillomania at least. Recent developments in pharmacotherapy for trichotillomania indicate that N-acetylcysteine, a glutamate modulator, is another viable treatment option that reduces hair-pulling behavior and urges (Grant et al. 2009), although studies of its efficacy in younger samples have yet to be completed. Patients whose comorbidities appear to be primary or in whom the comorbid symptoms (e.g., amotivation in depression) would be likely to interfere with delivery of more active forms of treatment would likely need to be referred to address the comorbid disorder first. Patients who are not highly motivated for treatment but otherwise appear likely to benefit from it are typically given the full range of options and an assessment of which would be most likely to require a good deal of their time and attention. As yet, however, there are no empirically supported protocols that have proven effective at enhancing motivation in trichotillomania or related problems per se, although motivational interviewing has been employed to address this issue for a host of psychiatric problems (Miller and Rollnick 2002). At this stage, a clinician's job is to present the choices to the family and to inform them of the likely consequences of their choices, then let the family decide what is in their best interest and in the best interest of the child.

REFERENCES

American Psychiatric Association: Diagnostic and Statistical Manual of Mental Disorders, 4th Edition. Washington, DC, American Psychiatric Association, 1994

American Psychiatric Association: Diagnostic and Statistical Manual of Mental Disorders, 4th Edition, Text Revision. Washington, DC, American Psychiatric Association, 2000

Bloch MH, Landeros-Weisenberger AL, Dombrowski P, et al: Systematic review: pharmacological and behavioral treatment for trichotillomania. Biol Psychiatry 62:839–846, 2007

Byrd MR, Richards DF, Hove G: Treatment of early onset hair pulling as a simple habit. Behav Modif 26:400–411, 2002

Christenson GA, Mackenzie TB, Mitchell JE, et al: A placebo-controlled, double-blind crossover study of fluoxetine in trichotillomania. Am J Psychiatry 148:1566–1571, 1991

Conners CK, Sitarenios G, Parker JD, et al: The Revised Conners' Parent Rating Scale (CPRS-R): factor structure, reliability, and criterion validity. J Abnorm Child Psychol 26:257–268, 1998

Cooper LD, Aronson L, Balsam PD, et al: Duration of signals for intertrial reinforcement and nonreinforcement in random control procedures. J Exp Psychol Anim Behav Process 16:14–26, 1990

Deckersbach T, Rauch S, Buhlman U, et al: Habit reversal versus supportive psychotherapy in Tourette's disorder: a randomized controlled trial and predictors of treatment response. Behav Res Ther 44:1079–1090, 2006

Diefenbach GJ, Tolin DF, Hannan S, et al: Trichotillomania: impact on psychosocial functioning and quality of life. Behav Res Ther 43:869–884, 2005

Flessner CA, Woods DW, Franklin ME, et al: The Milwaukee Inventory for Styles of Trichotillomania—Child Version (MIST-C): initial development and psychometric properties. Behav Modif 31:896–918, 2007

Flessner C, Conelea CA, Woods DW, et al: Styles of pulling in trichotillomania: exploring differences in symptom severity, phenomenology, and functional impact. Behav Res Ther 46:345–357, 2008

Flessner C, Penzel F, Keuthen N: Current treatment practices for children and adults with trichotillomania: consensus among experts. Cogn Behav Pract 17:290–300, 2010

Franklin ME, Tolin DF: Treating Trichotillomania: Cognitive Behavioral Therapy for Hair Pulling and Related Problems. New York, Springer Science and Business Media, 2007

Franklin ME, Flessner CA, Woods DW, et al: The Child and Adolescent Trichotillomania Impact Project: descriptive psychopathology, comorbidity, functional impairment, and treatment utilization. J Dev Behav Pediatr 29:493–500, 2008

Franklin ME, Rae A: Does case complexity actually matter? Impact of comorbidity on CBT outcomes in pediatric trichotillomania. Presented at the New Research Findings Seminar "Treatment of Habit Disorders in Adults and Children" (G Keijsers, Chair) at the World Congress of Behavioral and Cognitive Therapies, June 2010

Goodman WK, Price LH, Rasmussen SA, et al: The Yale-Brown Obsessive Compulsive Scale, I: development, use, and reliability. Arch Gen Psychiatry 46:1006–1011, 1989a

Goodman WK, Price LH, Rasmussen SA, et al: The Yale-Brown Obsessive Compulsive Scale, II: validity. Arch Gen Psychiatry 46:1012–1016, 1989b

Grant JE, Odlaug BL, Kim SW: N-Acetylcysteine, a glutamate modulator, in the treatment of trichotillomania. Arch Gen Psychiatry 66:756–763, 2009

Green B: The Children's Global Assessment Scale in clinical practice: an empirical evaluation. J Am Acad Child Adolesc Psychiatry 33:1158–1164, 1994

Hanna GL: Trichotillomania and related disorders in children and adolescents. Child Psychiatry Hum Dev 27:255–268, 1997

Kendall PC, Gosch E, Furr JM, et al: Flexibility within fidelity. J Am Acad Child Adolesc Psychiatry 47:987–993, 2008

Keuthen NJ, Wilhelm S, Deckersbach T, et al: The Skin Picking Scale: scale construction and psychometric analyses. J Psychosom Res 50:337–341, 2001

King RA, Scahill L, Vitulano LA: Childhood trichotillomania: clinical phenomenology, comorbidity, and family genetics. J Am Acad Child Adolesc Psychiatry 34:1451–1459, 1995

Kovacs M: The Children's Depression Inventory (CDI). Psychopharmacol Bull 21:995–998, 1985

Lerner J, Franklin ME, Meadows EA, et al: Effectiveness of a cognitive behavioral treatment program for trichotillomania: an uncontrolled evaluation. Behav Ther 29:157–171, 1998

Lewin AB, Piacentini J, Flessner CA, et al: Depression, anxiety, and functional impairment in children with trichotillomania. Depress Anxiety 26:521–527, 2009

March JS, Parker JD, Sullivan K, et al: The Multidimensional Anxiety Scale for Children (MASC): factor structure, reliability, and validity. J Am Acad Child Adolesc Psychiatry 36:554–565, 1997

Miller WR, Rollnick S: Motivational Interviewing: Preparing People for Change. New York, Guilford, 2002

Rapp JT, Miltenberger RG, Long ES, et al: Simplified habit reversal treatment for chronic hair pulling in three adolescents: a clinical replication with direct observation. J Appl Behav Anal 31:299–302, 1998

Reeve EA, Bernstein GA, Christenson GA: Clinical characteristics and psychiatric comorbidity in children with trichotillomania. J Am Acad Child Adolesc Psychiatry 31:132–138, 1992

Rothbaum BO: The behavioral treatment of trichotillomania. Behav Psychother 20:85–90, 1992

Rothbaum BO, Ninan PT: The assessment of trichotillomania. Behav Res Ther 32:651–662, 1994

Shaffer D, Gould MS, Brasic J, et al: A children's global assessment scale (CGAS). Arch Gen Psychiatry 40:1228–1231, 1983

Sheehan DV, Sheehan KH, Shytle RD, et al: Reliability and validity of the Mini International Neuropsychiatric Interview for Children and Adolescents (MINI-KID). J Clin Psychiatry 71:313–326, 2010

Silverman WK, Albano AM: Anxiety Disorders Interview Schedule for DSM-IV: Child Version. San Antonio, TX, Psychological Corporation, 1996

Storch EA, Merlo LJ, Larson MJ, et al: Impact of comorbidity on cognitive-behavioral therapy response in pediatric obsessive-compulsive disorder. J Am Acad Child Adolesc Psychiatry 47:583–592, 2008

Swedo SE, Leonard HL, Rapoport JL, et al: A double-blind comparison of clomipramine and desipramine in the treatment of trichotillomania (hair pulling). N Engl J Med 321:497–501, 1989

Tolin DF, Franklin ME, Diefenbach GJ: Cognitive-behavioral treatment of pediatric trichotillomania: an open trial, in Trichotillomania: Theory and Treatment. Symposium presented at the 31st Congress of the European Association of Behavioral and Cognitive Therapies, Maastricht, The Netherlands, September 2002

Tolin DF, Franklin ME, Diefenbach GJ, et al: Pediatric trichotillomania: descriptive psychopathology and an open trial of cognitive behavioral therapy. Cogn Behav Ther 36:129–144, 2007

Tolin DF, Diefenbach GJ, Flessner CA, et al: The Trichotillomania Scale for Children: development and validation. Child Psychiatry Hum Dev 39:331–349, 2008

Vitulano LA, King RA, Scahill L, et al: Behavioral treatment of children and adolescents with trichotillomania. J Am Acad Child Adolesc Psychiatry 31:139–146, 1992

Weissman MM, Prusoff BA, Thompson WD: Social adjustment by self-report in a community sample and in psychiatric outpatients. J Nerv Ment Dis 166:317–326, 1978

Woods DW: Premonitory Urge for Tics Scale (PUTS): initial psychometric results and examination of the premonitory urge phenomenon in youths with tic disorders. J Dev Behav Pediatr 26:397–403, 2005

Woods DW, Flessner C, Franklin ME, et al: Understanding and treating trichotillomania: what we know and what we don't know. Psychiatr Clin North Am 29:487–501, 2006

Wright HH, Holmes GR: Trichotillomania (hair pulling) in toddlers. Psychol Rep 92:228–230, 2003

ASSESSMENT OF TRICHOTILLOMANIA, PATHOLOGICAL SKIN PICKING, AND STEREOTYPIC MOVEMENT DISORDER

Nancy J. Keuthen, Ph.D.

Jedidiah Siev, Ph.D.

Hannah Reese, Ph.D.

The assessment of trichotillomania, pathological skin picking (PSP), and stereotypic movement disorder (SMD) presents an array of challenges to the practicing clinician. Issues exist regarding diagnostic classification, limited availability of assessment instruments (and variable psychometric properties for those scales that do exist), and changes in symptom presentation both within and across patients over time.

We wish to express our thanks to Amanda Allen and Elizabeth Loerke for their assistance in chapter preparation.

Different assessment instruments capture different dimensions of these disorders, including satisfaction of diagnostic criteria, symptom severity, disorder "styles," idiographic behavioral triggers and reinforcers, and associated psychosocial impairment. Given the potentially embarrassing nature of some of these symptoms (e.g., pubic hair pulling or skin picking), it is possible that different assessment methods (e.g., clinician vs. self-report measures) may yield discrepant clinical information although designed to evaluate the same aspect of the disorder. Accordingly, it is advisable to use multi-instrument, multimethod assessments as a best practice approach whenever possible, to ensure comprehensive, valid assessments both at baseline and throughout treatment. The absence of standardized assessment protocols for these disorders also argues for the utilization of multiple assessment instruments, when feasible, to optimize communication among treating professionals.

Selection of an assessment battery will depend on several factors. These include the purpose of the assessment (e.g., disorder diagnosis, benchmarking severity or impairment, or detailed characterization of the clinical picture) as well as the availability of professional resources (e.g., clinician expertise in instrument administration and time allotted for assessment) and the patient profile (e.g., comorbid clinical diagnoses and ability to complete scales or monitoring logs). The specific nature of the clinical setting (e.g., evaluation vs. treatment clinic) and the type of treatment (e.g., psychopharmacology vs. psychosocial treatment) will also factor into instrument choice. For instance, in a screening clinic, a diagnostic module may be used to determine disorder occurrence warranting subsequent treatment referral. In a treatment clinic, some combination of clinician-administered severity measures, self-rated scales, and "collateral" scale administration or behavioral observation may be selected to evaluate illness severity, depending on available clinician resources, patient capacity to perform ratings, and the involvement of significant others. For more focused cognitive-behavioral treatments, functional analysis interviews by the therapist coupled with patient monitoring of the target behavior plus its antecedents and consequences are warranted for the development of a tailored intervention for the specific patient.

When conducting an initial comprehensive assessment, the clinician should assess highly comorbid disorders (e.g., anxiety and mood disorders, substance abuse disorders), because the presence of these conditions may impact choice of treatment(s) and course of improvement. For example, the co-occurrence of severe depression may require targeted mood treatment prior to, or concurrent with, treatment of the presenting behavior problem. We also recommend assessment of other body-focused repetitive behaviors (BFRBs), given frequent covariation with one another. When comorbid BFRBs share similar reinforcement mechanisms, it is important to ensure that reduced occurrence of one behavior is not accompanied by increased occurrence of another dysfunctional behavior.

Needless to say, serial assessment throughout treatment is critical to evaluate changes in symptom severity, associated psychosocial impairment, and symptom profile. It is important to recognize that both quantitative and qualitative variability in symptoms occur over time even in the absence of intervention, because occurrence of the problem behaviors is determined by exposure to triggering stimuli. For example, student hair pullers often reduce pulling behavior during the summer months in the absence of academic stress and diminished involvement in sedentary computer activity. Similarly, picking behavior can worsen for women in the premenstrual part of the month due to acne breakouts from hormonal changes. Thus, the clinician should be thoughtful about the timing and duration of assessment periods, to ensure that assessment outcomes accurately represent overall behavioral severity and symptom picture. It is useful to gather several consecutive data points when possible for the most accurate representation of the clinical picture.

In this chapter, we focus primarily on the more formal assessment instruments for these disorders, including available diagnostic modules, clinician-administered instruments, and self- and parent-rated scales. Other existing assessment methods include self-monitoring, photographs and measurement of secondary physical damage, collection of removed tissue, functional analysis interviews, and observation by others. As with all assessment approaches, advantages and disadvantages exist for all of these methods. We first briefly discuss the general methods of assessment that apply across the disorders, before reviewing the formal assessment instruments specific to each disorder.

GENERAL ASSESSMENT APPROACHES

Self-Monitoring

Self-monitoring of symptoms and related variables can provide data for a functional analysis of behavior as well as assess the frequency and intensity of target behaviors at baseline and during treatment. Additionally, it can enhance awareness of the target behavior and related stimuli and decrease severity as a function of behavioral reactivity. The validity and utility of self-monitored data are directly contingent on compliance with recording. Self-monitoring is a time- and labor-intensive endeavor that requires considerable commitment on the part of the patient. The focus for self-monitoring can include occurrence of the problem behavior or, alternatively, urges, precursor motor behavior (such as touches or looks in trichotillomania or PSP), or cognitive behaviors (e.g., thoughts that specific hairs do not belong or the skin needs to be made smooth). Successful efforts to resist execution of the problem behavior can also be monitored. In some cases, as with stereotypic movements in individuals with comorbid mental retardation, the patient may lack the capacity to perform self-monitoring.

Photographic Assessment and Physical Measurement

When physical stigmata result from the problem behaviors (such as hair loss with trichotillomania and skin excoriation with PSP), photographic assessment and physical measurement of affected areas can potentially be useful. Twohig and colleagues (Twohig and Woods 2001; Twohig et al. 2006) used photographs as primary treatment outcome measures by having independent evaluators rate photographs for degree of tissue damage from PSP. These approaches, however, may not provide valid assessments when multiple body sites are involved at different times secondary to tissue damage or specific areas have been sensitized from prior behavior. These measures also are not feasible when private body areas are involved. Additionally, hair regrowth with behavioral abstinence may be delayed depending on the stage of the hair growth cycle; thus, hair regrowth may not always reflect behavioral change. Additionally, hair regrowth may not occur at all if the hair follicles have been severely damaged by prior pulling. Last, these problems can be accompanied by considerable shame, and the patient may prefer not to reveal the affected areas to the clinician.

Collection of Removed Tissue

Similarly, collection of removed tissue (e.g., extracted hair or picked skin) can be utilized to index behavioral severity. This method is not possible, however, when the patient lacks sufficient awareness of his or her behavior for tissue collection and in cases in which the tissue is ingested upon removal. Although some patients report that this approach is helpful, use of this method should first be discussed with the patient, because some may experience it as punitive.

Functional Analysis Interviews

Clinicians may conduct functional analysis interviews during which they query the patient about the unique antecedents and consequences to their problem behavior. Psychoeducation from the clinician during this process may facilitate greater awareness on the part of the patient of his or her unique behavioral triggers (e.g., situations, moods, physical sensations, motor movements, and cognitions) and reinforcers (e.g., the reduction of uncomfortable emotions or sensations or the occurrence of positive emotions or sensations). Given the lowered awareness that accompanies the habit-like style of tricho-

tillomania and PSP, self-monitoring by the patient is often necessary to identify the full complement of behavioral antecedents and consequences.

Observation by Others

Behavioral monitoring by significant others (e.g., parents, teachers, or caregivers) may be applicable with younger children or patients with intellectual deficits. This is only feasible with behaviors that are visible to others and when the
significant other has the time and skills to routinely observe the behavior.
When the behavior occurs with a high frequency, time-sampling methods may
be employed.

   We now review the instruments available for more formal assessment of
these disorders and their accompanying psychometric properties. We also
present unique considerations that impact assessment for each disorder.

TRICHOTILLOMANIA

Of the three disorders, trichotillomania arguably has the largest selection of
assessment instruments with known psychometric properties. Several newer
instruments assessing trichotillomania "styles" in adults and children, plus a
child self-report instrument with a parallel parent version, are welcome additions to the field. Despite recent developments, however, the assessment of
trichotillomania still remains limited. Psychometric study of several older clinician-administered instruments indicates that they lack suitability for routine use in the assessment of trichotillomania. The only published diagnostic
module was developed in accordance with DSM-III-R (American Psychiatric
Association 1987) criteria. A revision of this module has been utilized in research, but it lacks psychometric study. The self-report scales for adults and
children/parents assessing severity, disorder style, and psychosocial impairment have the most psychometric rigor at the present time.

   From a diagnostic standpoint, it is noteworthy that the current diagnostic
criteria for trichotillomania (DSM-IV-TR; American Psychiatric Association
2000) have been challenged as too restrictive given the absence of empirical
differences between pullers who do and do not endorse Criteria B and C (Stein
et al. 2010). Thus, similar treatments may be appropriate even with failure to
fully satisfy diagnostic criteria. In addition, the boundaries between trichotillomania and similar disorders remain unclear. It has been suggested that trichotillomania, not surprisingly, may be characterized as an SMD (Stein et al.
2008). Further empirical study of this question is clearly warranted.

   In the following subsections, we describe the available assessment instruments for trichotillomania by category and comment on their psychometric
properties (or lack thereof).

Diagnostic Modules

Trichotillomania Diagnostic Interview

The Trichotillomania Diagnostic Interview (TDI; Rothbaum and Ninan 1994) is a semistructured interview modeled after the Structured Clinical Interview for DSM-III-R (SCID; Spitzer et al. 1987). It consists of three-point item ratings assessing the DSM-III-R diagnostic criteria for trichotillomania. To ensure conformity with the DSM-IV-TR criteria for trichotillomania, a revision of the TDI (the TDI-R) was developed in the Trichotillomania Clinic and Research Unit at Massachusetts General Hospital/Harvard Medical School. In the TDI-R, Item 4 was modified to state, "Do you experience an increasing sense of tension before pulling out the hair, or when attempting to resist the behavior?" In addition, the question "Does your hair pulling cause you significant distress or impairment in social, occupational, or other important areas of functioning?" was added. Psychometric data are lacking for both the TDI and the TDI-R.

Clinician-Rated Measures

National Institute of Mental Health Trichotillomania Severity Scale and Trichotillomania Impairment Scale

The National Institute of Mental Health Trichotillomania Severity Scale (NIMH-TSS; Swedo et al. 1989) is a five-item, clinician-rated scale assessing pulling frequency (both on the previous day and during the past week), urge intensity, urge resistance, subjective distress, and interference with daily activities. Four items are rated from 0 (none) to 5 (most severe) and the final item is rated from 0 to 4. A total score is calculated by summing all the item scores.

The NIMH-TSS has reported sensitivity to changes in symptom severity (Lerner et al. 1998; Ninan et al. 2000; Swedo et al. 1989; Tolin et al. 2007). Interrater reliability for individual scale items and the total scale score varies across studies (Diefenbach et al. 2005; Stanley et al. 1999). There is evidence of concurrent validity with self-reported measures of trichotillomania severity (number of hairs pulled and time spent pulling) and other clinician-rated measures (Diefenbach et al. 2005; Stanley et al. 1999). Internal consistency ratings, however, have not been acceptable (Diefenbach et al. 2005; Stanley et al. 1999).

The NIMH Trichotillomania Impairment Scale (NIMH-TIS; Swedo et al. 1989) is a clinician-rated scale with a single global impairment score from 0 (absent) to 10 (severe). Ratings are based on severity of alopecia, time spent pulling or hiding damage, ability to control pulling, interference, and distress.

Similar to the NIMH-TSS, psychometric data for the NIMH-TIS are limited. Interrater reliability scores have been adequate (Stanley et al. 1999). Good concurrent validity has been reported with self-reported trichotillomania severity measures (Stanley et al. 1999) as well as clinician-rated measures (Diefenbach et al. 2005). The NIMH-TIS is sensitive to changes in trichotillomania impairment with treatment (e.g., Swedo et al. 1989).

Psychiatric Institute Trichotillomania Scale

The Psychiatric Institute Trichotillomania Scale (PITS; Winchel et al. 1992) is a semistructured instrument with a guided interview format consisting of six items assessing pulling sites, duration, resistance, interference, distress, and severity. Items are rated on an eight-point (0–7) scale, with anchors provided for each response rating. A total score is calculated by summing all of the individual items. Higher scores reflect greater symptom severity.

Interrater agreement is acceptable for most scale items, with moderate to good interrater agreement for total scale scores; however, internal consistency is below minimally acceptable standards (Diefenbach et al. 2005; Stanley et al. 1999). Finally, concurrent validity has been demonstrated between PITS item and total scores with self-report of overall trichotillomania severity, duration of pulling, and number of hairs extracted (Stanley et al. 1999) as well as with other clinician-rated scales and a self-report scale (Diefenbach et al. 2005). A criticism of this scale is that the definition of severity levels from the item response anchors appears somewhat arbitrary (Rothbaum and Ninan 1994).

Yale-Brown Obsessive Compulsive Scale—Trichotillomania

The Yale-Brown Obsessive Compulsive Scale—Trichotillomania (Y-BOCS-TTM; Stanley et al. 1993) is an adaptation of the Yale-Brown Obsessive Compulsive Scale (Y-BOCS; Goodman et al. 1989), a 10-item scale for rating the severity of obsessions and compulsions in obsessive-compulsive disorder. In the Y-BOCS-TTM, the phrase "thoughts about hair-pulling" replaces "obsessions" in the first five scale items, and the word "hair-pulling" replaces "compulsions" in the last five scale items. The instrument yields a total score and two subscale scores (Target Thoughts and Target Behaviors).

Psychometric evaluation indicates that this modification of the Y-BOCS has limited reliability and validity for assessing trichotillomania symptom severity. Item scores have been non-normally distributed for several items, especially those assessing hair-pulling-related thoughts (Stanley et al. 1993). Estimates of internal consistency for total and subscale scores have ranged from adequate to unacceptable (Stanley et al. 1993, 1999). Interrater reliabilities for individual items and summary scores have similarly ranged from excellent to poor (Stanley et al. 1993, 1999). Although test-retest correlation coefficients are statistically significant for the total scale and Target Thoughts subscale, they only approach significance for the Target Behaviors subscale

(Stanley et al. 1993). Although concurrent validity was demonstrated for total Y-BOCS-TTM scale scores with the Anxiety Disorders Interview Schedule—Revised (DiNardo and Barlow 1988) severity ratings of trichotillomania and self-monitored time spent thinking about trichotillomania, nonsignificant correlations were reported with self-monitored number of hairs extracted and time spent pulling hair (Stanley et al. 1993). Y-BOCS-TTM total scores did appear to be sensitive to changes in treatment when compared with self-reported number of hairs pulled (Stanley et al. 1993).

Self-Report Measures

Cues Checklist

The Cues Checklist (Mackenzie et al. 1995) is a 339-item self-report checklist of behavioral cues, including locations, activities, objects, feeling states, and circumstances. Patients who had one of three primary disorders—obsessive-compulsive disorder ($n=60$), bulimia nervosa ($n=61$), or trichotillomania ($n=75$)—were asked to identify those scale items that "if encountered" would "elicit or worsen" their "symptoms." Principal components analysis identified four rotated components. Trichotillomania patient scores were higher than the other two groups on Component 3, which consisted of sedentary activities. The total Cues Checklist score for the trichotillomania group correlated with duration of illness but not age at onset. Stepwise discriminant analysis correctly diagnosed all trichotillomania patients in the original study on the basis of their Cues Checklist scores.

Scores on the Cues Checklist can be useful for planning treatment, especially psychosocial intervention. Identification of specific cues (whether sedentary activities or uncomfortable feeling states) can focus the treatment by matching treatment strategies to specific cues. Whereas The Milwaukee Inventory for Subtypes of Trichotillomania—Adult Version (MIST-A) and The Milwaukee Inventory for Styles of Trichotillomania—Child Version (MIST-C) identify pulling styles, the Cues Checklist identifies the specific behavioral or emotional cues consistent with those styles.

Massachusetts General Hospital Hairpulling Scale

The Massachusetts General Hospital Hairpulling Scale (MGH-HPS; Keuthen et al. 1995) is a brief, self-report instrument for the assessment of hair-pulling severity. Trichotillomania-relevant items were adopted from the Y-BOCS, with "hairpulling" substituted for "compulsion." Y-BOCS items assessing obsessions were replaced with items assessing pulling urges. The scale consists of seven items (frequency and intensity of urges, ability to control urges, frequency of hair pulling, resistance to and control over hair pulling, and associated distress) rated on a severity scale ranging from 0 to 4.

The scale is homogeneous, with good internal consistency (Diefenbach et al. 2005; Keuthen et al. 1995, 2007a), excellent test-retest reliability (O'Sullivan et al. 1995), good convergent and divergent validity (Diefenbach et al. 2005; O'Sullivan et al. 1995), and sensitivity to change in symptoms (O'Sullivan et al. 1995). Exploratory factor analysis revealed two separate scale factors of "severity" and "resistance and control" (Keuthen et al. 2007a).

Milwaukee Inventory for Subtypes of Trichotillomania— Adult Version

The MIST-A (Flessner et al. 2007b) is a 15-item, self-rated instrument developed from a large (N=1,697) Internet study of self-reported hair pullers. Exploratory factor analysis revealed two distinct factors measuring "focused" pulling (10 items) and "automatic" pulling (5 items); this factor structure was also supported by subsequent confirmatory factor analysis. The MIST-A consists of two separate scales with items rated from 0 ("not true of my hair pulling") to 9 ("true for all of my hair pulling").

The Focused and Automatic Pulling Scales both have demonstrated good internal consistency with two separate samples (Flessner et al. 2007b). Correlations with awareness of pulling, self-report of physical or mental anxiety prior to pulling, pulling to achieve symmetry or a specific bodily sensation, and the Depression, Anxiety, and Stress Scales indicate good construct validity for both the Focused and Automatic Pulling Scales. Lastly, the two scales are weakly correlated, suggesting good discriminant validity.

Milwaukee Inventory for Styles of Trichotillomania—Child Version

The MIST-C (Flessner et al. 2007a) is a 25-item scale developed to assess styles of hair pulling in children and adolescents. Exploratory factor analysis on an earlier version of the scale revealed two factors: focused pulling (21 items) and automatic pulling (4 items). Items are rated from 0 ("not true for any of my pulling") to 9 ("true for all of my pulling"), with individual item scores summed separately for focused and automatic pulling scores. Higher scores indicate greater focused or automatic pulling.

Psychometric evaluation in a sample of youth (n=164) revealed good (α=0.80) to excellent (α=0.90) internal consistency for the automatic and focused pulling scales, respectively. Construct validity was demonstrated by correlating scores on the separate subscales with relevant items (e.g., proportion of time children reported awareness of pulling and self-reported physical and mental anxiety) from the Trichotillomania Impact Survey for Children (M.E. Franklin, C. Flessner, D.W. Woods, unpublished, 2006) and other scales. Discriminant validity was demonstrated by the nonsignificant correlation between the focused and automatic pulling scales.

Trichotillomania Scale for Children

The Trichotillomania Scale for Children (TSC; Tolin et al. 2008) is a 12-item scale assessing hair-pulling severity, distress, and impairment, with parallel child (TSC-C) and parent (TSC-P) versions. It was developed on an Internet sample of children endorsing criteria for trichotillomania (N=113) and their parents (N=132), coupled with 41 parent–child dyads from an outpatient clinic setting. Principal components analysis revealed two components labeled "severity" (five scale items) and "distress/impairment" (seven scale items).

Internal consistency was demonstrated to be adequate to good for total and subscale scores on the TSC-C and TSC-P for both the Internet (α= 0.76–0.85) and clinic (α=0.71–0.83) samples. Adequate test-retest reliability was reported in the clinic sample for total and subscale scores on the TSC-C (r=0.81–0.89) and the TSC-P (r=0.70–0.97). Parent/child agreement assessed by Pearson correlations between TSC-C and TSC-P scores was adequate to high for the Internet sample but only moderate, yet significant, for the clinic sample. Convergent validity was generally demonstrated for TSC-C score correlations with other trichotillomania indices of severity. TSC-P scores for the Internet sample correlated with other parent-rated measures of trichotillomania severity. However, TSC-P scores for the clinic sample had less significant correlations with child- and interviewer-rated measures of trichotillomania severity.

PATHOLOGICAL SKIN PICKING

The assessment of PSP, like trichotillomania, has a range of clinician-administered and self-report scales as well as an unpublished diagnostic module. The clinician-administered instruments have, for the most part, not received adequate psychometric scrutiny. As is the case for trichotillomania, the patient-rated measures for PSP have the strongest psychometric support.

From the perspective of diagnostic classification, it bears mentioning that PSP is not currently recognized as a formal disorder in DSM-IV-TR. In current practice, PSP is variously diagnosed as obsessive-compulsive disorder, impulse-control disorder not otherwise specified, or SMD, when the picking behavior is not symptomatic of another primary psychiatric disorder (e.g., body dysmorphic disorder or delusional disorder) or dermatological disorder (e.g., scabies).

Diagnostic Modules

Although PSP currently lacks a formal diagnostic category within DSM-IV-TR, Keuthen and colleagues have developed a brief diagnostic interview for the assessment of clinically significant skin picking. The Keuthen Diagnostic Inventory for Skin Picking (K-DISP) is a six-item semistructured interview modeled after the SCID (First et al. 2002). The diagnostic criteria applied by Keuthen and colleagues closely mirror the DSM-IV-TR diagnostic criteria for trichotillomania. Accordingly, the instrument assesses for 1) recurrent skin picking that results in noticeable tissue damage; 2) increasing tension before picking or when attempting to resist; 3) pleasure, gratification, or relief when picking; and 4) significant distress or impairment as a result of the picking. The picking can also not be better accounted for by a medical or skin condition or other psychological disorder. To date, no psychometric data have been published on the K-DISP.

Clinician-Rated Measures

Yale-Brown Obsessive Compulsive Scale Modified for Neurotic Excoriation

The NE-YBOCS (Arnold et al. 1999) was modeled after the Y-BOCS (Goodman et al. 1989), the gold standard clinician-rated measure of obsessive-compulsive disorder symptom severity. The NE-YBOCS includes 10 items. Items 1–5 assess the urges to pick or thoughts about picking. Items 6–10 assess the picking behavior. Similar to the original Y-BOCS, each item is rated on a 0–4 scale, and total scores range from 0 to 40. Formal psychometric evaluation of the NE-YBOCS has not been performed. It has, however, demonstrated good test-retest reliability (Spearman correlation = 0.83) and good construct validity when compared with other outcome measures in one treatment study (Grant et al. 2007).

Skin Picking Treatment Scale

The Skin Picking Treatment Scale (SPTS; Simeon et al. 1997) is a clinician-rated measure of PSP also modeled after the Y-BOCS (Goodman et al. 1989). It consists of five items that assess the urge to pick, time spent picking, picking severity, the degree of control over picking, and interference due to picking. Again, similar to the original Y-BOCS, each item is rated on a 0–4 scale. Thus, total scores range from 0 to 20. No psychometric data have been published on the SPTS, although it has been used in two treatment outcome studies (Bloch et al. 2001; Simeon et al. 1997).

Self-Report Measures

Skin Picking Scale

The Skin Picking Scale (SPS; Keuthen et al. 2001b) is a self-report measure that was also modeled after the Y-BOCS (Goodman et al. 1989). It includes six items assessing the frequency and intensity of the urges to pick; time spent picking;and interference, distress, and avoidance due to skin picking. Again, similar to the original Y-BOCS, each item is rated on a 0–4 scale. Thus, total scores range from 0 to 24. The SPS has moderate internal consistency (α = 0.80) and good construct validity (Keuthen et al. 2001b). A cutoff score of seven or above was shown to reliably distinguish between self-injurious skin pickers and non-self-injurious skin pickers. The SPS has also demonstrated sensitivity to change with treatment (Keuthen et al. 2007b).

Skin Picking Impact Scale

The Skin Picking Impact Scale (SPIS; Keuthen et al. 2001a) is a brief measure of the emotional (e.g., "I feel embarrassed because of my skin picking"), social (e.g., "My relationships have suffered because of my skin picking"), and behavioral (e.g., "There are some things I can't do because of my skin picking") consequences of skin picking. The measure includes 10 items. Respondents rate the degree to which each item applies to them in the previous week on a scale from 0 to 5. Thus, total scores range from 0 to 50. The SPIS has high internal consistency (α = 0.93) and good construct validity (Keuthen et al. 2001a). Similar to the SPS, a cutoff score of seven or more was shown to reliably distinguish between self-injurious skin pickers and non-self-injurious skin pickers. The SPIS has also demonstrated sensitivity to change with treatment (Keuthen et al. 2007b).

Habit Questionnaire

The Habit Questionnaire (Teng et al. 2002) is a self-report measure developed to screen for the presence of a range of problematic BFRBs, including skin picking, skin biting, skin scratching, nail biting, and mouth chewing. Respondents rate the frequency and duration of each endorsed behavior as well as any associated impairment, injury, medical attention, or intervention. They are also asked whether the behavior occurs only under the influence of alcohol or other substances and whether they have ever been diagnosed with any of the following comorbid conditions: obsessive-compulsive disorder, Tourette syndrome, autism, Asperger's syndrome, or a developmental disability. Teng and colleagues specified criteria for a BFRB as a behavior that occurs more than five times a day for 4 weeks or longer and results in impairment in functioning, injury, medical attention, or intervention. The Habit Questionnaire demonstrated moderate test-retest reliability in a sample of 105 undergraduate students (Phi = 0.69).

Skin Picking Symptom Assessment Scale

The Skin Picking Symptom Assessment Scale (SP-SAS; Grant et al. 2007) is a 12-item measure of skin picking modeled after existing measures of kleptomania (Grant and Kim 2002) and pathological gambling (Kim et al. 2001). Respondents rate each symptom over the past week on a 0–4 scale. Thus, total scores range from 0 to 48. The SP-SAS has demonstrated adequate test-retest reliability (Spearman correlation = 0.74) and satisfactory construct validity when compared with other outcome measures in one treatment outcome study (Grant et al. 2007).

Milwaukee Inventory for the Dimensions of Adult Skin Picking

The Milwaukee Inventory for the Dimensions of Adult Skin Picking (MIDAS; Walther et al. 2009) is an instrument that measures two types of skin picking: automatic picking and focused picking. The 12-item measure includes 6 items assessing automatic picking (e.g., "I am usually not aware of picking my skin during the picking episode") and 6 items assessing focused picking (e.g., "I pick my skin when I am experiencing a negative emotion such as stress, anger, frustration, or sadness"). Each item is rated on a 1 ("not true of any of my skin picking") to 5 ("true for all of my skin picking") scale. Thus, scores on each subscale range from 6 to 30. The MIDAS has adequate internal consistency (automatic subscale: $\alpha = 0.77$; focused subscale: $\alpha = 0.81$) and good construct validity (Walther et al. 2009).

STEREOTYPIC MOVEMENT DISORDER

The formal assessment of SMD is perhaps the most challenging given its varied presentation, common comorbidities, and blurred diagnostic boundaries with other disorders. There are few scales that measure stereotypy, and most of those that do were developed for use with developmentally or intellectually disabled individuals. Furthermore, scales that measure stereotypy and repetitive behaviors are typically lacking validation and standardization (e.g., Goldman et al. 2009; Symons et al. 2005).

The psychometric properties of the available measures are not well characterized in any population but are virtually unknown in adults without autism spectrum disorders or mental retardation. Hence, the clinician working with normally developed adults is faced with using existing measures as "proxy methods" to the extent that they appear to have face validity and utility for evaluating SMD in their patients. Existing checklists of common stereotypies may prove useful to the clinician who requires a comprehensive way of identifying specific behaviors for the design and implementation of a psychosocial intervention. Similarly, measures of overall severity may be appropriate to monitor outcome with psychosocial or pharmacological treatment.

In what follows, we review several scales that clinicians may find useful in assessing stereotypy. We sought to select the measures that have the most clinical utility and are widely available. We have not included several unpublished or ad hoc rating systems (e.g., Berkson et al. 1995; Wehmeyer 1994), checklists that are not easily obtained (e.g., Bodfish et al. 1995), or systems of observational coding (e.g., Campbell 1985; Goldman et al. 2009). We also have not included measures used exclusively for children (e.g., Nisonger Child Behavior Rating Form [Aman et al. 1996]).

Finally, considering that stereotypic behavior is characteristic of various disabilities and disorders, many measures of severe developmental or intellectual disability include some items to assess stereotypy (e.g., Aberrant Behavior Checklist [Aman et al. 1985]; Gilliam Autism Rating Scale–2 [Gilliam 2006]; Diagnostic Assessment for the Severely Handicapped–II [Matson 1995]). In order to facilitate the selection of measures most likely to have utility in assessing SMD, we review only those instruments primarily focused on stereotypic behavior or that have been used in studies of SMD. All of the instruments described here are designed for those adults (e.g., caregivers or parents) who provide care for the individual with SMD.

Because stereotypic movement is common and associated with various clinical features, a careful and thorough assessment is crucial. In a recent study of children with SMD but without autism spectrum disorders, sensory impairment, intellectual disability, or self-injurious behavior, prior misdiagnosis was normative (Freeman et al. 2010). More than half of the children were incorrectly referred for tics, and others were referred for autism spectrum disorders, compulsions, and epilepsy.

Diagnosis/Classification

The hallmark of SMD is a pattern of repetitive, seemingly nonfunctional and driven behavior. Stereotypies may be evident in individuals with cognitive deficits, developmental disorders, sensory deprivation, or autism spectrum disorders and in normally developing adults (e.g., Castellanos et al. 1996; Muthugovindan and Singer 2009; Rapp and Vollmer 2005). SMD is not formally diagnosed when the behavior is better accounted for by obsessive-compulsive, tic, or pervasive developmental disorders or by trichotillomania. Indeed, many behaviors can be labeled "stereotypies," and there is no definitive consensus about where to draw a diagnostic boundary (Rapp and Vollmer 2005). To our knowledge, there are no published diagnostic modules available for the assessment of SMD.

One classification system for stereotypies was developed by Muthugovindan and Singer (2009). They distinguished between *primary stereotypies*, which occur in children with healthy development, and *secondary stereotypies*, which are associated with another disorder (including sensory or neurological impairment). Moreover, they identified three types of primary stereotypies: common, head nodding, and complex motor. Common stereotypies include habits such as nail biting and thumb sucking. Individuals with repetitive head nodding need to be assessed for several other diagnoses, including bobble-head doll syndrome, spasmus nutans, Sandifer syndrome, congenital nystagmus, jactatio capitis nocturna, and oculomotor apraxia (Muthugovindan and Singer 2009). Complex motor stereotypies (e.g., flapping or finger writhing) can also occur in developmentally delayed or autistic children. Thus, care is necessary to distinguish primary from secondary stereotypies, particularly because the motor behaviors can be similar (e.g., Loh et al. 2007)

Clinician- and Caregiver-Rated Measures

Stereotypy Severity Scale

The Stereotypy Severity Scale (SSS; Miller et al. 2006) is a modified version of the Yale Global Tic Severity Scale (Leckman et al. 1989), a clinician-rated instrument. The SSS is revised to measure stereotypic movements instead of tics. The SSS has a motor component and a global impairment rating. The former comprises ratings of stereotypic movements to assess number (rated 0–3), frequency (0–5), intensity (0–5), and interference (0–5). These ratings are similar to the Yale Global Tic Severity Scale tic ratings, except that the number rating scale is modified and there is no rating for complexity. The global impairment rating ranges from 0 to 50. No known psychometrics are available for the SSS.

Stereotypy Linear Analog Scale

The Stereotypy Linear Analog Scale (SLAS; Miller et al. 2006) was used to capture dimensions similar to those measured by the SSS. Miller et al. (2006) asked parents to mark on a 10-cm line their children's recent stereotypic behavior from 0 ("the best it has ever been") to 10 ("the worst it has ever been"). Parents were instructed to consider number, frequency, intensity, and interference (i.e., the elements of the motor component of the SSS). No known psychometrics are available for the SLAS.

Repetitive Behavior Scale—Revised

The Repetitive Behavior Scale—Revised (RBS-R; Bodfish et al. 2000) is a 43-item measure of behaviors characteristic of individuals with autism spectrum disorders. Raters indicate frequency/interference on a four-point scale, from "behavior does not occur" (0) to "behavior occurs and is a severe problem" (3). The RBS-R yields six conceptual subscales, including Stereotypic Behavior and Self-Injurious Behavior.

Factor analysis of the measure in a sample of children and adults with autism spectrum disorders revealed a five-factor solution that retained the two aforementioned subscale labels, although the specific items were not identical (Lam and Aman 2007). Lam and Aman (2007) found high internal consistency for both the Stereotypic Behavior subscale (which includes six items) and the Self-Injurious Behavior subscale (which includes eight items). Interrater reliability appeared adequate in one sample but poor for the Stereotypic Behavior subscale in a sample with more severe mental retardation. Although the RBS-R was developed and tested primarily in autistic samples, researchers have used it to examine children with SMD but no autism spectrum or intellectual disorder (Freeman et al. 2010).

Stereotyped Behavior Scale

The Stereotyped Behavior Scale (SBS; Rojahn et al. 1997, 2000) was developed as a measure of stereotypic behavior in adolescents and adults with mental retardation. It consists of 24 items that assess both frequency (six-point scale) and severity (four-point scale) of stereotyped behaviors that are "conspicuous to the average person, and appear unusual, strange, or inappropriate. They are voluntary, idiosyncratic actions that repeat or recur."

The authors emphasized that the SBS is not intended as a diagnostic instrument for movement disorders because it does not differentiate the function or cause of the stereotyped behavior (Rojahn et al. 1997). Internal consistency was high, and the instrument was sensitive (i.e., identifying most individuals who, in fact, exhibited stereotyped behavior). In addition, validity and both test-retest and interrater reliability were good, although item-level reliability was lower. Normative data for the measure are presented by Rojahn et al. (2000).

Behavior Problems Inventory

The Behavior Problems Inventory (BPI-01; Rojahn et al. 2001) is a 52-item measure designed to assess stereotypic, self-injurious, and aggressive/destructive behavior in developmentally disabled adolescents and adults. The SBS was originally developed separately and was later incorporated into the larger measure, the BPI-01. We discuss the BPI-01 primarily because the Self-Injurious subscale includes items that may represent stereotypic behavior in the context of SMD.

The BPI-01 presents a list of specific behavior problems, and the rater indicates which ones have been observed during the past 2 months. Each item is rated on frequency (never, monthly, weekly, daily, hourly) and severity (no problem, slight, moderate, severe). The BPI-01 yields separate subscale scores for stereotypic, self-injurious, and aggressive/destructive behavior. (Of note, there have been several iterations in the development of this instrument, including revisions, additions, and translations.)

Stereotyped behavior is defined in the BPI-01 as behavior looking "unusual, strange, or inappropriate to the average person. They are voluntary acts that occur repeatedly in the same way over and over again, and they are characteristic for that person. However, they do NOT cause physical damage." The stereotyped behavior subscale comprises 25 items (24 specific items and 1 "Other" category). Hence, the stereotyped behavior subscale scores range from 0 to 100 for frequency and 0 to 75 for severity. *Self-injurious behavior* (SIB) is defined in the BPI-01 as behavior causing "damage to the person's own body…SIBs occur repeatedly in the same way over and over again, and they are characteristic for that person." The SIB scale has 15 items, including an "Other" category, and scores therefore range from 0 to 60 for frequency and 0 to 45 for severity.

Psychometric evaluations of the BPI-01 indicate that overall the measure is valid and reliable, with adequate internal consistency (e.g., Gonzalez et al. 2009; Rojahn et al. 2001). Nevertheless, there is some variability in the performance of the subscales across studies and samples. For example, interrater reliability for the Stereotypy subscale was low in the Gonzalez et al. (2009) study, and internal consistency was low for the Self-Injurious Behavior scale in that study as well as another (Rojahn et al. 2010). Moreover, the utility of the SBS and BPI-01 in assessing SMD is unclear; we are not aware of any data on the psychometric properties of either measure in a sample without developmental or intellectual disabilities.

Repetitive and Restricted Behaviour Scale

The Repetitive and Restricted Behaviour Scale (RRB; Bourreau et al. 2009) is a 35-item measure of behaviors seen in individuals with autism spectrum disorders and yields four subscales: Sensorimotor Stereotypies, Reaction to Change, Restricted Behaviours, and Modulation Insufficiency. Each item is rated on a five-point scale indicating "the degree of expression of each behaviour" from 0 ("the behaviour is never expressed") to 4 ("the behaviour is very characteristic of the individual and very severely expressed"). The RRB is intended to be completed by professional caregivers who have observed the target individual across several daily situations.

In the validation study, interrater reliability for the subscales was high (intra-class correlation coefficient=0.84–0.94) and for individual items ranged from moderate to excellent (weighted κ=0.46–0.90). However, all participants in the validation study were diagnosed with an autism spectrum disorder. Therefore, the utility and properties of the measure in individuals without developmental disabilities is not known, and further research is necessary to examine it as a potential assessment measure for use in SMD.

CONCLUSION

In this chapter, we sought to underscore the multitude of challenges that confront the clinician in the assessment of trichotillomania, PSP, and SMD. To start, it bears mentioning that our conceptualization of these problems has been rapidly evolving. This has resulted in changing diagnostic criteria (except for PSP, which yet lacks formal recognition in DSM-IV-TR) and unclear boundaries among disorders. The more formal assessment instruments for these disorders have historically often been adopted prior to appropriate psychometric scrutiny. On a more positive note, however, we now have several newer instruments that address long-standing assessment needs. Taken together, it is incumbent on individual clinicians to be thoughtful about the timing of their assessments and the selection of their instruments and methods. It is not feasible to establish standard assessment protocols for these disorders without specifying the purpose of the assessment, the clinical setting, available resources, and the specific population. Whenever possible, however, we strongly encourage the use of a multi-instrument, multimethod best-practice approach to provide the most comprehensive evaluation possible.

REFERENCES

Aman MG, Singh NN, Stewart AW, et al: The Aberrant Behavior Checklist: a behavior rating scale for the assessment of treatment effects. Am J Ment Defic 89:485–491, 1985

Aman MG, Tassé MJ, Rojahn J, et al: The Nisonger CBRF: a child behavior rating form for children with developmental disabilities. Res Dev Disabil 17:41–57, 1996

American Psychiatric Association: Diagnostic and Statistical Manual of Mental Disorders, 3rd Edition, Revised. Washington, DC, American Psychiatric Association, 1987

American Psychiatric Association: Diagnostic and Statistical Manual of Mental Disorders, 4th Edition, Text Revision. Washington, DC, American Psychiatric Association, 2000

Arnold LM, Mutasim DF, Dwight MM, et al: An open clinical trial of fluvoxamine treatment of psychogenic excoriation. J Clin Psychopharmacol 19:15–18, 1999

Berkson G, Gutermuth L, Baranek G: Relative prevalence and relations among stereotyped and similar behaviors. Am J Ment Retard 100:137–145, 1995

Bloch MR, Elliott M, Thompson H, et al: Fluoxetine in pathologic skin-picking: open-label and double-blind results. Psychosomatics 42:314–319, 2001

Bodfish JW, Crawford TW, Powell SB, et al: Compulsions in adults with mental retardation: prevalence, phenomenology, and comorbidity with stereotypy and self-injury. Am J Ment Retard 100:183–192, 1995

Bodfish JW, Symons FJ, Parker DE, et al: Varieties of repetitive behavior in autism: comparisons to mental retardation. J Autism Dev Disord 30:237–243, 2000

Bourreau Y, Roux S, Gomot M, et al: Validation of the Repetitive and Restricted Behaviour Scale in autism spectrum disorders. Eur Child Adolesc Psychiatry 18:675–682, 2009

Campbell M: Timed Stereotypies Rating Scale. Psychopharmacol Bull 21:1082, 1985

Castellanos FX, Ritchie GF, Marsh WL, et al: DSM-IV stereotypic movement disorder: persistence of stereotypies of infancy in intellectually normal adolescents and adults. J Clin Psychiatry 57:116–122, 1996

Diefenbach GJ, Tolin DF, Crocetto J, et al: Assessment of trichotillomania: a psychometric evaluation of hair-pulling scales. J Psychopathol Behav Assess 27:169–178, 2005

DiNardo PA, Barlow DH: The Anxiety Disorders Interview Schedule—Revised. Albany, State University of New York at Albany, Center for Stress and Anxiety Disorders, 1988

First MB, Spitzer RL, Gibbon M, et al: Structured Clinical Interview for DSM-IV-TR Axis I Disorders, Research Version, Patient Edition (SCIP-I/P). New York, Biometrics Research, 2002

Flessner CA, Woods DW, Franklin ME, et al: The Milwaukee Inventory for Styles of Trichotillomania—Child Version (MIST-C): initial development and psychometric properties. Behav Modif 31:896–918, 2007a

Flessner CA, Woods DW, Franklin ME, et al: The Milwaukee Inventory for Subtypes of Trichotillomania—Adult Version (MIST-A): development of an instrument for the assessment of "focused" and "automatic" hair pulling. J Psychopathol Behav Assess 30:20–30, 2007b

Freeman RD, Soltanifar A, Baer S: Stereotypic movement disorder: easily missed. Dev Med Child Neurol 52:733–738, 2010

Gilliam J: GARS-2: Gilliam Autism Rating Scale, 2nd Edition. Austin, TX, Pro-Ed, 2006

Goldman S, Wang C, Salgado MW, et al: Motor stereotypies in children with autism and other developmental disorders. Dev Med Child Neurol 51:30–38, 2009

Gonzalez ML, Dixon DR, Rojahn J, et al: The Behavior Problems Inventory: reliability and factor validity in institutionalized adults with intellectual disabilities. J Appl Res Intellect Disabil 22:223–235, 2009

Goodman WK, Price LH, Rasmussen SA, et al: The Yale-Brown Obsessive-Compulsive Scale, I: development, use, and reliability. Arch Gen Psychiatry 46:1006–1011, 1989

Grant JE, Kim SW: An open-label study of naltrexone in the treatment of kleptomania. J Clin Psychiatry 63:349–356, 2002

Grant JE, Odlaug BL, Kim SW: Lamotrigine treatment of pathological skin picking: an open-label study. J Clin Psychiatry 68:1384–1391, 2007

Keuthen NJ, O'Sullivan RL, Ricciardi JN, et al: The Massachusetts General Hospital (MGH) Hairpulling Scale, 1: development and factor analyses. Psychother Psychosom 64:141–145, 1995

Keuthen NJ, Deckersbach T, Wilhelm S, et al: The Skin Picking Impact Scale (SPIS): scale development and psychometric analysis. Psychosomatics 42:397–403, 2001a

Keuthen NJ, Wilhelm S, Deckersbach T, et al: The Skin Picking Scale: scale construction and psychometric analysis. J Psychosom Res 50:337–341, 2001b

Keuthen NJ, Flessner CA, Woods DW, et al: Factor analysis of the Massachusetts General Hospital Hairpulling Scale. J Psychosom Res 62:707–709, 2007a

Keuthen NJ, Jameson M, Loh R, et al: Open-label escitalopram treatment for pathological skin picking. Int Clin Psychopharmacol 22:268–274, 2007b

Kim SW, Grant JE, Adson DE, et al: Double-blind naltrexone and placebo comparison study in the treatment of pathological gambling. Biol Psychiatry 49:914–921, 2001

Lam KSL, Aman MG: The Repetitive Behavior Scale–Revised: independent validation in individuals with autism spectrum disorders. J Autism Dev Disord 37:855–866, 2007

Leckman JF, Riddle MA, Hardin MT, et al: The Yale Global Tic Severity Scale: initial testing of a clinician-rated scale of tic severity. J Am Acad Child Adolesc Psychiatry 28:566–573, 1989

Lerner J, Franklin ME, Meadows EA, et al: Effectiveness of a cognitive behavioral treatment program for trichotillomania: an uncontrolled evaluation. Behav Ther 29:157–171, 1998

Loh A, Soman T, Brian J, et al: Stereotyped motor behaviors associated with autism in high-risk infants: a pilot videotape analysis of a sibling sample. J Autism Dev Disord 37:25–36, 2007

Mackenzie TB, Ristvedt SL, Christenson GA, et al: Identification of cues associated with compulsive, bulimic, and hair-pulling symptoms. J Behav Ther Exp Psychiatry 26:9–16, 1995

Matson JL: The Diagnostic Assessment for the Severely Handicapped–II. Baton Rouge, LA, Scientific Publishers, 1995

Miller JM, Singer HS, Bridges DD, et al: Behavioral therapy for treatment of stereotypic movements in nonautistic children. J Child Neurol 21:119–125, 2006

Muthugovindan D, Singer H: Motor stereotypy disorders. Curr Opin Neurol 22:131–136, 2009

Ninan PT, Rothbaum BO, Marsteller FA, et al: A placebo-controlled trial of cognitive-behavioral therapy and clomipramine in trichotillomania. J Clin Psychiatry 61:47–50, 2000

O'Sullivan RL, Keuthen NJ, Hayday CF, et al: The Massachusetts General Hospital (MGH) Hairpulling Scale, 2: reliability and validity. Psychother Psychosom 64:146–148, 1995

Rapp JT, Vollmer TR: Stereotypy I: a review of behavioral assessment and treatment. Res Dev Disabil 26:527–547, 2005

Rojahn J, Tassè MJ, Sturmey P: The stereotyped behavior scale for adolescents and adults with mental retardation. Am J Ment Retard 102:137–146, 1997

Rojahn J, Matlock ST, Tassé MJ: The Stereotyped Behavior Scale: psychometric properties and norms. Res Dev Disabilities 21:437–454, 2000

Rojahn J, Matson JL, Lott D, et al: The Behavior Problems Inventory: an instrument for the assessment of self-injury, stereotyped behavior, and aggression/destruction in individuals with developmental disabilities. J Autism Dev Disord 31:577–588, 2001

Rojahn J, Rowe EW, Macken J, et al: Psychometric evaluation of the Behavior Problems Inventory-01 and the Nisonger Child Behavior Rating Form with children and adolescents. J Ment Health Res Intellect Disabil 3:28–50, 2010

Rothbaum BO, Ninan PT: The assessment of trichotillomania. Behav Res Ther 32:651–662, 1994

Simeon D, Stein DJ, Gross S, et al: A double-blind trial of fluoxetine in pathologic skin picking. J Clin Psychiatry 58:341–347, 1997

Spitzer RL, Williams JBW, Gibbon M, et al: Structured Clinical Interview for DSM-III-R (SCID). New York, Biometrics Research Division, New York State Psychiatric Institute, 1987

Stanley MA, Prather RC, Wagner AL, et al: Can the Yale-Brown Obsessive Compulsive Scale be used to assess trichotillomania? A preliminary report. Behav Res Ther 31:171–177, 1993

Stanley MA, Breckenridge JK, Snyder AG, et al: Clinician-rated measures of hair pulling: a preliminary psychometric evaluation. J Psychopathol Behav Assess 21:157–170, 1999

Stein DJ, Flessner CA, Franklin M, et al: Is trichotillomania a stereotypic movement disorder? An analysis of body-focused repetitive behaviors in people with hair-pulling. Ann Clin Psychiatry 20:194–198, 2008

Stein DJ, Grant JE, Franklin ME, et al: Trichotillomania (hair pulling disorder), skin picking disorder, and stereotypic movement disorder: toward DSM-V. Depress Anxiety 27:611–626, 2010

Swedo SE, Leonard HL, Rapoport JL, et al: A double-blind comparison of clomipramine and desipramine in the treatment of trichotillomania (hair pulling). N Engl J Med 321:497–501, 1989

Symons FJ, Sperry LA, Dropik PL, et al: The early development of stereotypy and self-injury: a review of research methods. J Intellect Disabil Res 49:144–158, 2005

Teng EJ, Woods DW, Twohig MP, et al: Body focused repetitive behavior problems: prevalence in a nonreferred population and differences in perceived somatic activity. Behav Modif 26:340–360, 2002

Tolin DF, Franklin ME, Diefenbach GJ, et al: Pediatric trichotillomania: descriptive psychopathology and an open trial of cognitive behavioral therapy. Cogn Behav Ther 36:129–144, 2007

Tolin DF, Diefenbach GJ, Flessner CA, et al: The Trichotillomania Scale for Children: development and validation. Child Psychiatry Hum Dev 39:331–349, 2008

Twohig MP, Woods DW: Habit reversal as a treatment for chronic skin picking in typically developing adult male siblings. J Appl Behav Anal 34:217–220, 2001

Twohig MP, Hayes SC, Masuda A: A preliminary investigation of acceptance and commitment therapy as a treatment for chronic skin picking. Behav Res Ther 44:1513–1522, 2006

Walther MR, Flessner CA, Conelea CA, et al: The Milwaukee Inventory for the Dimensions of Adult Skin Picking (MIDAS): initial development and psychometric properties. J Behav Ther Exp Psychiatry 40:127–135, 2009

Wehmeyer ML: Factors related to the expression of typical and atypical repetitive movements of young children with intellectual disability. International Journal of Disability, Development, and Education 41:33–49, 1994

Winchel RM, Jones JS, Molcho A, et al: The Psychiatric Institute Trichotillomania Scale (PITS). Psychopharmacol Bull 28:463–476, 1992

Part 3

TREATMENT

Chapter 9

COGNITIVE-BEHAVIORAL THERAPY FOR PEDIATRIC TRICHOTILLOMANIA

Mayumi Okada Gianoli
David F. Tolin, Ph.D., ABPP

The treatment outcome literature on trichotillomania remains underdeveloped, particularly regarding the treatment of children and adolescents. However, cognitive-behavioral therapy (CBT) appears to be one of the more promising treatments for this disorder (Bloch et al. 2007; Stein et al. 1999). CBT for child and adolescent disorders, as for adults, emphasizes the influence of and interaction among cognitions, behavior, affect, and the social environment in maintaining maladaptive behavior. In this chapter, we describe the process and application of CBT for the treatment of pediatric trichotillomania (elementary school–age children and older).

Modern CBT approaches contain multiple intervention strategies, which can be applied in a modular fashion (Franklin and Tolin 2007; Penzel 2003; Woods and Miltenberger 2001). The specific interventions for adult and pediatric trichotillomania include 1) rapport building and information gathering; 2) psychoeducation; 3) awareness training using self-monitoring; 4) stimulus control; 5) competing response training; and 6) relapse prevention strategies. Although a course of treatment typically follows this general sequence (with significant overlap between modules), the skilled clinician may draw from these principles at various times throughout the treatment. We discuss each intervention in the following sections.

RAPPORT BUILDING AND INFORMATION GATHERING

As with CBT for other disorders, therapy for pediatric trichotillomania begins by establishing a trusting therapeutic relationship between the child and the therapist. Depending on the child's age and developmental level, it may be appropriate and comforting to the child to include the parent during this first session. When the therapist is working with adults, rapport building is almost always done in the context of gathering information about their problems. However, for younger children, it may be necessary to ease them into therapy more gradually by asking and talking about their hobbies or engaging in simple activities or games.

A functional analysis is developed to facilitate treatment planning, based on the premise that pulling behaviors are maintained by their antecedents and consequences. This fine-grained information about the functional context of the child's pulling behavior is typically obtained using a detailed interview, during which detailed information about antecedents (a chain of events that lead up to the pulling behavior), the pulling behaviors, and post-pulling events are collected. Antecedents may be conceptually divided into early triggers and pre-pulling events. In gathering information about the early triggers, it is helpful to ask the child to start at the point of pulling and work backward to the earliest antecedents he or she can identify. Possible early triggers include (but are certainly not limited to) setting, specific activities, posture, thoughts, emotions, physiological sensations, arousal level, and urges to pull. Having developed an understanding of the early antecedents, the therapist can ask the child to describe events that immediately precede the problem behavior. These pre-pulling events can include preparatory grooming-like behaviors (e.g., touching hair); tactile or visual cues; change in thoughts, feelings, or physiological sensations; and urges to pull.

The next area of assessment is the problem behavior itself and the events that follow it. A complete assessment of these events may include a detailed description of the behavior; any change in thoughts, feelings, or physiological sensations during and immediately following the behavior; visual behaviors such as looking at the pulled hair; tactile behaviors such as touching or rolling the pulled hair; oral behaviors such as biting or eating the hair; the method of discarding the pulled hair; and any changes in thoughts, feelings, or physiological sensations during and immediately following the post-pulling behaviors.

Such fine details are important for two main reasons. First, specific information about pulling-related thoughts, feelings, and behaviors can be employed in the service of psychoeducation and model building (discussed later), as well as to "normalize" symptoms in the course of psychoeducation (e.g., many children and parents are surprised to learn that eating hair is common among people with trichotillomania). Second, this information is particularly useful in tailoring intervention strategies to match the specific needs of the child (e.g., which strategies should be emphasized and which can be de-emphasized or eliminated).

PSYCHOEDUCATION

In addition to helping the child and his or her parents to better understand the nature of his or her trichotillomania, psychoeducation also sets the stage for developing effective intervention strategies. We suggest providing a schematic diagram of the biopsychosocial model (Franklin et al. 2006) when providing information about trichotillomania. An example of a schematic diagram is shown in Figure 9–1. When working with children and adolescents, the clinician should use age-appropriate language and focus on those elements that are most critical to the intervention (see Figure 9–2 for an example of a child's completed diagram). The diagram in total may seem overwhelming for many young children; therefore, we emphasize the need to explain each part of the model slowly using developmentally appropriate language and soliciting questions along the way. It will also be helpful to incorporate the information that the clinician has gathered, to illustrate how the child's pulling is related to internal and external triggers as well as to alterations in internal sensations that may be reinforcing the problem behavior. Orientation to the biopsychosocial model depicted in Figure 9–2 might go as follows:

> You've done a really good job in helping me to understand what may be going on. Although I don't know for sure why you started pulling in the first place, I think I may be able to explain why you keep pulling. As you can see in this diagram [*show the diagram to child*], over time, your brain has decided that when you are in certain situations or doing certain activities or thinking something or feeling something in particular, you're going to pull. So, whenever you are in that situation, like doing homework at the kitchen table, your brain tells you that it's time to pull. Sometimes you'll get that "I want to pull, I have to pull" feeling; sometimes you won't notice that feeling but your brain will just get your fingers to start doing it. And when you pull, it changes the way you feel. Maybe it distracts you from that stressed and bored feeling that you get from having to do homework. Or maybe pulling makes your scalp feel good for a little bit. Either way, your brain learns that pulling is good because it either makes the bad feelings go away or makes the good feelings come. Of course, these feelings don't last very long, so maybe a few minutes or seconds after you pull your hair—and in fact, in time you end up feeling guilty and embarrassed—your brain tells you that you need to pull again to get that good feeling back or to make that bad feeling go away, again for just a little bit. See, that's why it's hard to stop pulling after one hair.

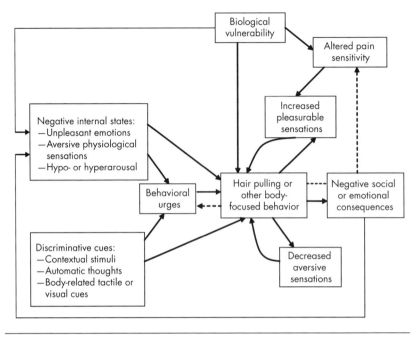

FIGURE 9–1.   A proposed biopsychosocial model of trichotillomania.

Source.   Adapted from Franklin et al. 2006.

Successful treatment is predicated on a collaborative working relationship with the child. Therefore, it is critical that the child and his or her parents be well informed about trichotillomania and its treatment. Prior to the start of treatment, the therapist should set aside ample time to solicit questions from the child and parents. Children and their family members should be reminded that there are no "dumb" questions and that many people have what they perceive to be "strange" concerns only to find out that their questions are actually quite common. Some common questions involve the reasons for hair pulling, the epidemiology of trichotillomania in young people, the likelihood of immediate and long-term recovery, the likelihood of successful hair regrowth, and the relationship between trichotillomania and obsessive-compulsive disorder. Clinicians should use the information in this book, along with child- and parent-friendly language and examples, to answer as many questions as possible.

AWARENESS TRAINING USING SELF-MONITORING

Awareness training is typically initiated early in the therapy. One technique used to improve awareness is self-monitoring. A filled-out self-monitoring form is shown in Figure 9–3.

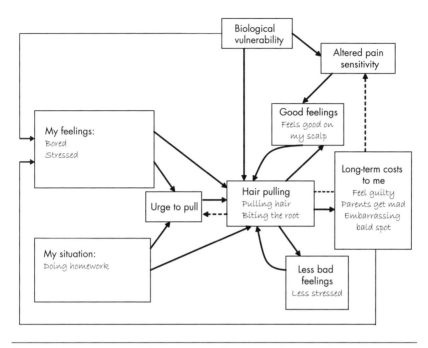

FIGURE 9–2. A modified functional analysis diagram for children with trichotillomania.

Self-monitoring may be introduced to the child with an analogy about the need to carefully examine a phenomenon before deciding how to respond appropriately. Sports metaphors work especially well for this purpose (e.g., football coaches and players watch films to identify their opponent's tendencies before designing plays that may work against the opponent). Self-monitoring may also be presented to the child as a way of "playing detective" or "spying on trich" to determine when it may strike next so that clinician and child can better anticipate its next move and "catch trich in the act." These metaphors should always be tailored to the interests and developmental level of the individual. It is also important to feed back to the child the information that he or she provided during the assessment session. Orientation to self-monitoring may go as follows:

> When we talked last week, we noticed that you pull most often in the evening when you're doing your homework at the kitchen table. It usually starts after a few minutes of combing through your hair with your left hand first, and you find that hair that "feels wrong" right before you begin pulling. You've done a great job in helping me to understand some important things about your pulling pattern, but for us to figure out what would be most

Day/Date	Time	What I was doing & where	What I was thinking, feeling before pulling	Played with hair before pulling? (Y/N)	# hairs pulled	Consequence
Mon 3/1	3:45 pm	Doing homework at kitchen table	I hate this homework! Feeling frustrated	Yes	9	Distracted Felt calmer Got mad at self later
Mon 3/1	7:55 pm	Talking to my friend on the phone about the school project	I can't focus on what my friend is saying because my brothers are so loud! Annoyed; irritated	Yes	10	Felt like I could focus better Less irritated Felt nice

FIGURE 9–3.   Self-monitoring form for trichotillomania.

helpful for you to stop pulling, we need to try to understand it a little more. One of the best ways to do that is to begin keeping track of trich as it's happening, and that's why I want you to begin self-monitoring after our session today [*take out two self-monitoring sheets and hand one to child*]. I made this sheet for you so that you can record what you are thinking or feeling just before you start pulling. You can also write down if you were touching your hair before you started and how many hairs you pulled out that time.

It is important that the child understand the self-monitoring assignment. Using information about the child's last pulling episode, the therapist and child should spend some time completing a self-monitoring sheet together in session. This will help to clarify what the child is expected to do as he or she is asked to begin self-monitoring.

T: Just for practice, let's try to use this sheet to record what you remember about the last time you pulled. When was that?

C: Yesterday when I was doing my homework at the kitchen table.

T: Okay, let's write down yesterday's date in the "Day/Date" column. And "doing homework at the kitchen table" in the "What I was doing and where" column. Do you remember what time it was?

C: My brothers had just come home from soccer, so maybe 4?

T: Good. Let's write down "4 o'clock" in the "Time" column. Do you remember if you were touching your hair before the pulling started?

C: Yeah, I was combing through my hair.

T: And how were you feeling when you were doing that?

C: Um, kind of annoyed because I was reading this really boring book.

T: And what were you thinking about?

C: Just thinking or feeling like I was stupid and I hate math.

T: Okay. Let's get all that information down on your sheet. Do you remember if you felt any weird feelings, like on your fingers or your head, before you pulled your hair?

C: Yeah, I always get that tingly feeling on my head.

T: Okay, and how many hairs did you pull?

C: Maybe 10?

T: And how did you feel then?

C: I felt a little less frustrated, like it distracted me a little. But later on I got mad at myself when I realized how much I had pulled.

It is important to emphasize the benefits of monitoring pulling behavior as it is happening, rather than retrospectively. Not only does real-time monitoring improve the accuracy of the recorded information, but it also improves the child's awareness of the pulling habit. Furthermore, self-monitoring forms can serve as a form of stimulus control, because the child must stop pulling in order to retrieve his or her monitoring sheets. Self-monitoring may also be thought of as a form of competing response because it creates a behavior with the hands and fingers (writing) that is incompatible with pulling.

Saving pulled hairs is another technique that can improve awareness of pulling and also serve as a check for the child on the accuracy of self-monitoring. In this strategy, the child is asked to collect pulled hairs in an envelope and to bring this envelope to each of the subsequent treatment sessions. Although some children may find this technique uncomfortable, there are several reasons to include it. One of the benefits of saving pulled hairs is that it provides another objective measure of pulling. This may help in improving the accuracy of self-monitoring data, given that the child is made aware that the therapist will ask to inspect the sheets and the collected hairs. Placing the pulled hairs immediately into an envelope may also curtail some of the post-pulling behaviors that some children find reinforcing, such as rolling the hair between their fingers, carefully examining the pulled hair, rubbing the hair on their faces and lips, biting off the root, sticking the root to a piece of paper, or ingesting the hair. It is important to underscore that this technique is designed not to be embarrassing or humiliating but rather to serve these other purposes. Explaining how the hair will be used in session may also help to alleviate some concerns:

> During our session, as we look over the self-monitoring sheets, we're also going to open up the envelope to take a look at how many hairs are in there. We're going to look to see that the number of hairs in the envelope matches the number of hairs that you have written on your sheet, and then, after that, we will throw the envelope with the hairs in the trash. Then, we'll continue our session.

For some, this early awareness training sets the stage for successful implementation of stimulus control and competing response training. In these cases, the therapist should work with the child to graph the number of hairs pulled and then, using the self-monitoring sheets, look for any early signs of a pattern to pulling, such as location (e.g., desk at school), time of day, or consistent affective triggers (e.g., boredom). Efforts to self-monitor are praised effusively, especially during this early phase of treatment. Younger children may respond to external reinforcers for accuracy, such as colorful stickers to decorate their folders and monitoring sheets.

Some children (or parents) may be disappointed that they have continued to pull despite entering treatment. It may be important to remind these individuals that the purpose of self-monitoring is not necessarily to decrease the pulling behavior but rather to increase awareness of pulling and its context.

The clinician should examine the self-monitoring data to determine whether the child knows (or could be taught to know) in advance whether he or she might pull. Again, with younger children, we use analogies of "playing detective" or "spying on trich" to determine if the child is aware of any precursors to pulling (i.e., "Now that you've been doing a good job spying on trich, did you notice that there were certain places, times, or activities during which trich showed up?"). As part of the monitoring review, the therapist and the child quickly scan the collected hairs to see if the number of pulled hairs recorded on the monitoring sheet corresponds roughly to the amount of hair in the envelope. If there is much more hair in the envelope than was recorded, the clinician should inquire about whether each pulling episode was tracked, as well as about the placement of the envelope and the monitoring sheets. In cases in which the envelope may have been more readily accessible (compared with the monitoring sheets, resulting in more hair in the envelope than was recorded), the child should be reinforced for his or her efforts to save hairs, but the therapist should specify that the envelope should be moved further away, giving the child an incentive to break the rhythm of pulling by getting up, retrieving the envelope and the folder, and recording the pulling episode immediately. On the contrary, if the number of recorded hairs greatly exceeds the amount in the envelope, it is important to inquire gently about the child's possible reluctance to place hairs in the envelope, inadequate planning (e.g., envelope kept in a much less accessible place), or previously undisclosed trichophagia (eating hair).

The clinician's task is more complicated when the child returns with partially complete or missing monitoring sheets. In such cases, a problem-solving approach is encouraged. It is not helpful to simply label this behavior as "noncompliance"; instead, as with other difficulties that these patients may experience, this too should be conceptualized as a problem that requires active participation from the therapist, the child, and his or her parents to solve. This discussion should begin by eliciting from the child his or her own account of why the monitoring task proved difficult and using this information to generate potential solutions together. When working with very young children, it is important to keep in mind that they often do not have the ability to monitor their behavior very carefully. Thus, it may be necessary to have the parents play a more active role in keeping track of pulling behaviors with these children.

Self-monitoring continues throughout the entire protocol, because changing the contingencies in response to observed patterns can sometimes lead to changes in the pulling pattern that must themselves be monitored and addressed. It may be useful to convey this idea using an analogy:

> When people are trying to get rid of mice in their homes, they plug up the big holes that they know the mice are using. But when they plug up those big holes, the mice may find other holes and begin using those or maybe

they'll even dig new holes. Closing the big holes is very helpful, but that's just the first step. We need to see what the mice will do next. The same thing applies to when we're trying to get rid of trich. We first figure out when trich happens the most, then when we take care of that, we need to watch and see where else trich will show up.

STIMULUS CONTROL

The concept of stimulus control is introduced early in the treatment. The rationale is as follows: Over time, pulling behavior becomes associated with a variety of internal and external contextual cues through classical conditioning (Azrin and Nunn 1973; Mansueto et al. 1997). Controlling the habit, therefore, may depend partly on controlling the context in which the behavior occurs; in other words, choosing different situations or changing the environment in some meaningful way may help to control the problem behavior. Both adults and children receiving CBT for trichotillomania have rated stimulus control to be one of the most helpful components of the treatment (Brady et al. 2005; Tolin et al. 2002).

Referring back to Figure 9–1, we note that contextual stimuli can be either internal or external. Internal cues for pulling may include hypo- or hyperarousal, physiological sensations, or negative cognitions (Christenson et al. 1993; Gluhoski 1995; Mansueto 1990). If internal contextual cues are identified, it may be useful to consider augmenting the basic protocol with additional strategies such as relaxation training or cognitive restructuring. External cues are frequently visual; many with trichotillomania report that their pulling is preceded by a visual scan of that region of the body. For example, a person with trichotillomania may look at his or her hair in the mirror searching for a hair that stands out in some way (e.g., is shorter than others, curly, damaged). Tactile sensations (e.g., sensations produced by the hair on the skin such as on the fingertips) may also precede the pulling. For example, individuals may run their fingers through their hair searching for hair that feels different (e.g., coarse, curly, damaged). Some have reported that this behavior is pleasurable in and of itself, suggesting that pre-pulling behavior may itself be positively reinforcing. Others have reported that pulling episodes often occur when in certain postures (proprioceptive cues), most often with the hand close to the site of pulling, such as leaning the head on the left hand while reading. Pulling can also be triggered when the person is in a specific location. Some pull exclusively in one location (e.g., on the couch in the living room), whereas others pull in a variety of locations but the behavior is worse in certain places. Similarly, activities can become associated with pulling. We often find that such activities contribute to hypo- or hyperarousal. Many children, for example, report pulling while studying or doing other forms of homework that they find stressful. They may also report pulling during tasks in which they feel impatient—for example, while waiting for e-mails or instant messages on the computer. Others tend to pull when they are understimulated, such as while watching television. It is important to keep in mind that the effect of any of these contextual cues may be modified by the presence of certain discriminative cues (factors that increase or decrease the likelihood of pulling). Therefore, it is not sufficient to know that the child typically pulls while watching television; the therapist must also ascertain the conditions under which this relationship is observed. For example, the child may report that he or she pulls in front of the television, but only when alone (i.e., the presence of others inhibits the relationship between TV watching and pulling). Another child may report that he or she pulls when doing homework but not when the assignment involves written work (i.e., activities that involve writing inhibit the relationship between homework and pulling). Discriminative cues, although subtle, may greatly moderate the effects of the contextual cues.

Stimulus control is used to minimize the person's exposure to stimuli that tend to trigger pulling, while maximizing his or her exposure to stimuli that tend to minimize pulling. The rationale may be presented as follows:

> Sometimes when we pull over and over again in one place or during a certain activity, just being in that place or doing that activity can make us want to pull. To make it easier to stop pulling, we may have to change something about that place or that activity. This idea works for other things besides trich too. See, I love to eat potato chips when I'm watching TV sitting in my favorite comfy chair. I've done it so much that it's become a habit. I know that I should stop eating those chips, but now, when I sit in that chair and turn the TV on, I just get really hungry for those chips. If I want to stop eating those chips, I may have to change something about it. I'm not about to give up my TV, but maybe instead of watching TV by myself, I can watch TV with my friends so that they can stop me from eating chips. Let's see if we can work together to figure out what kinds of small changes we can make to some of the situations that make you want to pull.

In the following discussion, we describe some specific stimulus control strategies.

Visual Cues

Intervention typically involves limiting the child's visual access to the area. For example, the parents might be encouraged to cover the child's bathroom mirror with newspaper. A patient who pulls hair from her legs or arms might be encouraged to wear long pants or long sleeves.

Tactile/Proprioceptive Cues

Children who are triggered by tactile cues should be encouraged to limit the touching of their hair or skin. Often, we will encourage patients to wear rubber fingertips or gloves on one or both hands, particularly in "high risk" situations such as watching TV. To counteract proprioceptive triggers, we will often encourage children to change positions, such as not resting their heads in their hands while doing homework.

Location Cues

When practical, exposure to high-risk locations should be minimized in the early stages of treatment. For example, a child who pulls while watching TV in the basement might be encouraged to watch TV in the family living room instead. When exposure cannot be minimized, we often introduce other forms of stimulus control into these locations to minimize the risk of pulling. For example, a patient who pulls while lying in bed might be encouraged to wear gloves to bed for this reason.

Activity Cues

We have, at times, encouraged young people to take a break from using instant-messaging software when such activity (particularly waiting for a reply) is strongly associated with pulling. However, pulling is often associated with activities that cannot reasonably be avoided; in such cases, we find it helpful to use gloves or other tactile sensation–reducing articles or to introduce negative discriminative cues such as those described in the following section.

Discriminative Cues

The therapist can introduce contextual cues that modify the relationship between the situation and the behavior. For many patients, pulling occurs only in private, when the person knows he or she will not be observed. Therefore, introducing the presence (or potential presence) of others may be a useful intervention. For example, an adolescent trichotillomania patient may not be able to avoid lying in her bed at night, but she may be persuaded to leave her bedroom door open in order to make the situation less private. Some patients benefit from visual reminders, left in high-risk areas, not to pull. Children in particular often enjoy making large "stop" signs to hang in the bedroom or bathroom or by the computer or television.

When stimulus control procedures are being implemented, it is important to identify the earliest possible point in the behavioral chain for intervention. The most common mistake in stimulus control (as well as competing response training) is to wait until the last minute to implement the procedures. By this point, the urge often has grown too strong for the child to manage. As Masters et al. (1987) noted, "Certain people seem to believe that the mark of self-control is the ability to withstand any and all temptation. In fact, it is far more correct to say that the mark of self-control is the ability to minimize temptation by early interruption of such behavioral chains" (pp. 451–452).

COMPETING RESPONSE TRAINING

One of the more commonly used components of CBT for trichotillomania is competing response training (CRT), which was first introduced by Azrin and Nunn (1973) as a component of habit reversal training, a general intervention for nervous habits and tics. The original rationale for habit reversal training posited that nervous habits persist partly because they operate outside conscious awareness. For some people with trichotillomania, their picking/pulling behaviors sometimes take place outside of awareness (e.g., unfocused pulling); however, in many cases, the person is quite aware of the behavior (Flessner et al. 2008).

CRT for trichotillomania often involves encouraging children to touch, squeeze, or play with objects when they feel an urge to pull. Many children with trichotillomania have found that playing with rubber "koosh" balls, perhaps because of the hairlike quality of the rubber "legs," is an effective competing response. There is virtually no limit to the number of possible CRT behaviors. What is critical is that the behavior is 1) easy for the person to implement and 2) motorically inconsistent with pulling. Other examples of CRT activities that have been effectively used include playing with clay or a ball of string; shelling peanuts; tying and retying one's shoes; playing with jewelry such as rings, necklaces, or bracelets; squeezing a "stress ball"; and grasping other objects such as a pencil, a book, or the steering wheel of a car. CRT activities do not necessarily require the person to have something to hold in his or her hands. Examples of "self-contained" CRT behaviors include making a fist and squeezing, putting one's hands into one's pockets, and sitting on one's hands. Regardless of the activity chosen, CRT begins by instructing the child to engage in the chosen activity whenever he or she feels an urge to pull. Over time, the child is taught to start engaging in his or her chosen CRT activity progressively earlier in the pulling sequence, with the ultimate goal being that the child learns to engage in competing behaviors before he or she is conscious of urges to pull in any situation that may trigger the urge to pull.

It is important to note that CRT goes beyond merely "keeping one's hands busy." Whereas stimulus control is designed as a preventive measure (i.e., it can be done at all times), CRT is intended to be used as a contingency for pulling urges and/or behavior. That is, these behaviors should be employed when the child is aware of pulling urges or is engaged in pulling or pre-pulling behavior. Following the principle of overcorrection, we generally recommend that the child engage in the competing behavior for 3 full minutes (although we recognize that children and adolescents may have difficulty complying with this instruction, in which case they are instructed to engage in the competing behavior for at least 30 seconds). The long-duration competing response is designed to allow the individual's urges to subside while he or she is engaging in the competing behavior. CRT demonstrates that if the child does not pull, his or her discomfort or urge will eventually subside. Thus, in addition to the behavioral aspect of CRT, from a cognitive perspective, CRT reinforces the idea that the child does not need to pull in order to reduce discomfort.

In this session, the therapist introduces the concept of CRT and provides the child with introductory exercises. Keep in mind that the initial goal is to simply have the child engage in the competing response exercise, not for the competing behavior to prevent pulling.

> During our last sessions, we talked about how your hair pulling usually goes, what kinds of situations tend to make you want to pull, and what do you get out of pulling. We've also worked on some ways to increase your own awareness of pulling, such as being more aware of where your hands are, what your fingers are doing, and so on. Now, let's start working on reducing the hair pulling itself. What I'm going to suggest may seem a bit strange, and it may be kind of inconvenient for you. But people seem to find this to be very helpful. So, I'm going to ask you to do something else with your hands whenever you find yourself pulling. We can pick any activity we want, as long as it's something that you can do easily and it's something that you can do for about 3 minutes. It also has to be something that you couldn't do if you were pulling your hair.

At this point, the therapist encourages the child to brainstorm ideas for their competing response behavior. Should they choose an activity that involves objects, it will be important to ask about the ease of obtaining and using the object at any given time. It may be necessary to help generate ideas for increasing accessibility to the object. For example, if the child decides to use a "stress ball," the therapist may begin by asking where the ball should be kept, and through direct or indirect suggestions recommend placing stress balls throughout the house to ensure easy access to a ball at any given time. In addition, a conversation about how the object will be used (e.g., the child will squeeze the stress ball tightly) may be helpful. Finally, a rationale for engaging in the competing response behaviors needs to be presented.

> I think that squeezing a stress ball is a great idea, especially now that we've talked about how you're going to leave the balls in the places that you're most likely to pull, such as the kitchen, the bathroom, and your bedroom. And another great thing about your idea is that you won't be able to pull your hair and squeeze the ball at the same time. Now, as I said before, I'm going to be asking you to keep squeezing the ball really tight for 3 minutes every time. Now, 3 minutes is a long time, but that's why this strategy is going to be so helpful. You see, you can beat the urge to pull without being 100% free of urges 100% of the time. A lot of times, all you need is to be able to get through that immediate period when the urges are really strong. By squeezing the ball for 3 minutes, what you're doing is making sure that you're squeezing long enough for the urge to come down to a level where you can resist it. Also, by doing this, you're going to be showing yourself that you don't need to pull for your urges to get better; if you hang in there and do something else besides pulling, your urges will come down anyway.

After the rationale has been presented, the therapist should model how to engage in CRT. Additionally, to ensure that the child understands what is to be expected, the therapist may choose to have the child mimic the therapist after the CRT sequence has been modeled once. To facilitate the process, the therapist can provide step-by-step directions.

> Let me show you how it will go [*place a stress ball on the desk*]. I have my stress ball here on the kitchen table, just like we agreed. Now, I'm going to start reading [*mimic reading*]. Now, I start combing through my hair with my left hand [*start combing through hair*], I find a hair that feels kind of coarse, one that I'd really like to pull. [*Remove hand from hair and picks up stress ball with the same hand.*] So now, I drop what I'm doing, grab the stress ball, and squeeze. And I'm going to hold it for 3 minutes. Now you try it. [*Place the stress ball in front of child.*]

RELAPSE PREVENTION STRATEGIES

The literature on long-term maintenance of gains following any treatment for trichotillomania is limited, but the data seem to indicate that the better a child does in the short term, the better he or she will do in the long term (Tolin et al. 2007). Thus, many of the clinical strategies that are used during acute treatment are also used to help patients remain well. There are, however, several techniques that specifically address maintenance. Borrowing from the research literature on substance abuse treatment, the aims of relapse prevention are to prevent the return of symptoms and to help patients get "back on track" if lapses occur (Parks et al. 2001).

Many patients, especially those who have made substantial progress in CBT for trichotillomania, often become alarmed at the prospect of having to fight the disorder "on their own" after the treatment course has been completed. To alleviate this specific concern, booster sessions are scheduled in advance (e.g., bimonthly sessions, monthly sessions followed by "check-ups" as needed). At the same time, later sessions emphasize how the child (and not the therapist) is credited for the progress that he or she has made through the use of identifying high-risk situations via careful self-monitoring, modifying the environment via stimulus control methods, and implementing habit reversal methods at the first sign of urges to pull. Therapists also emphasize the child's increased knowledge about trichotillomania, the theoretical foundation of CBT approaches, and how best to implement the treatment procedures. Children and adolescents seem to appreciate learning that they are now much more knowledgeable about these key issues than are many, if not most, mental health professionals. To help reinforce the belief that they are capable of handling any future "bumps in the road," therapists may consider asking them to recount how they were able to make progress on their trichotillomania and quiz them on what to do if they encounter new urges to pull. Every opportunity to reinforce their newfound knowledge should be used to allay concerns that the therapist or the clinic (or something/someone other than the child) was primarily responsible for the change. For younger children, therapists may choose to formalize the end of a treatment course by holding a graduation ceremony during the last session (see March and Mulle 1998).

By the time the latter stages of acute CBT have been reached, most patients are aware that many people with trichotillomania have at least some ongoing urges to pull and even actual pulling. The therapist should emphasize that the urge to pull should, however, no longer be a cause for alarm because the patient has now developed effective methods to deal with these urges. It may be helpful to review how he or she can go about using stimulus control and competing response training techniques when either the urge to pull or actual pulling has crept back in. Additionally, in preparing for a long-term battle against trichotillomania, there should be some psychoeducation about lapses (defined as temporary slipups in refraining from pulling and/or occurrence of intense urges) and relapses (a return to the old ways of managing urges to pull hair) as well as instructions for responding to occasional lapses by putting the treatment techniques into place.

As the active phase of CBT treatment comes to an end, it may be beneficial to devote some time to exploring how the trichotillomania may have "derailed" the patient in various areas of social functioning. For example, some children may have been "shy" about meeting new people or engaging in hobbies because of their trichotillomania. Given that continued functional impairment and avoidance are stressful and hence risk factors for the development of increased urges, pulling, and relapse, it may be beneficial to collaborate with the child to problem-solve issues related to reintegration.

INVOLVING PARENTS IN SESSIONS

It is frequently helpful to include the child's parents in sessions. As described by Kendall (2006), family members can serve as consultants, when they provide input regarding the nature of the problem; as co-clients, when they are viewed as contributing to aspects of the child's problems; or as collaborators, when they are asked to assist their child in implementing various aspects of the treatment program. In most sessions with children and adolescents, the preferred session structure is to work only with the child or the adolescent for approximately 40 minutes, then to invite the parents to join during the last 10–15 minutes. During this shared time (when the parents, the child, and the therapist are together), the child is asked to summarize for the parent what was covered in the session, explain the theoretical rationale for chosen procedures, and describe the assigned homework for the coming week. Next, the therapist checks in with the parents to see if there are any specific questions or issues they wish to raise. Such a structure is preferred because it simultaneously underscores the central role that the child must play in treatment and reinforces for parents that the treatment "belongs" to the child, with the parents in a supportive role.

Most children and adolescents whom we have seen experience significant distress or impairment in role functioning as a result of their hair pulling. They have described experiencing embarrassment and shame, social avoidance, and a host of problems that impact their functioning. However, for some young children, pulling appears to be only minimally disturbing, even though it is extremely difficult on their parents. In such cases, psycho-education about trichotillomania can be useful to assuage parents' anxieties about the child's future (such as his or her ability to make friends or succeed in school) or concerns that the parents might have "caused" the trichotillomania. It is also important to assist parents in recognizing that if the child is functioning well in school, has friends, and appears to be happy and unconcerned about the trichotillomania, he or she is unlikely to feel strong motivation to change this behavior and thus would likely exhibit low CBT compliance and outcome. If the child does not appear to be at all upset about the behavior, then it may not be the right time to initiate CBT. Of course, with young children, contingency management strategies for stimulating motivation to comply with CBT methods may be used, because many children do not fully appreciate the long-term implications of behavior and are more responsive to proximal rewards. However, when children are not at all bothered by their pulling or its consequences and are unwilling to engage in a treatment process to reduce a behavior that they do not see as problematic, the best strategy may be to delay treatment initiation.

EFFICACY OF COGNITIVE-BEHAVIORAL THERAPY FOR PEDIATRIC TRICHOTILLOMANIA

It is generally well accepted that CBT is efficacious for adult trichotillomania, at least in the short term (Bloch et al. 2007), although risk of relapse appears high after treatment discontinuation (Diefenbach et al. 2006; Lerner et al. 1998; Mouton and Stanley 1996).

By comparison, CBT for pediatric trichotillomania has received little empirical attention. In a preliminary open trial, Tolin et al. (2007) treated 22 children (77% female; mean age, 13 years) with a primary diagnosis of trichotillomania. CBT was divided into two phases. The first phase (active treatment) lasted 8 weeks and consisted of weekly individual CBT sessions as described in this chapter, plus some attention to additional strategies such as progressive muscle relaxation (Bernstein and Borkovec 1973) and cognitive restructuring (Beck 1995). The second phase (relapse prevention) consisted of four biweekly sessions, interspersed with brief (15- to 20-minute) telephone contacts with the therapist. In this phase, the emphasis was on reminding the child to employ previously learned strategies and to remain aware of pulling behaviors. During these sessions, the therapist reviewed the child's use of strategies and helped troubleshoot any problems that arose between visits. Results showed a significant decrease in trichotillomania severity over the course of treatment, with 77% of the intent-to-treat sample identified as treatment responders (much improved or very much improved). Of the 17 children classified as responders at the end of treatment (week 16), 4 (23.5%) had lost this designation during a 6-month follow-up period, suggesting relatively good maintenance of treatment gains.

In a subsequent randomized controlled trial, Franklin et al. (2007) assigned 24 children (67% female; mean age, 12 years) to the same CBT protocol as used in the open trial (Tolin et al. 2007) or to a minimal attention control condition (for ethical reasons, the minimal attention condition was 8 weeks long compared with 16 weeks for CBT). Results showed that children receiving CBT exhibited a significant decrease in trichotillomania severity at the 8- and 16-week time points, with 50% of the intent-to-treat sample identified as "excellent responders" (minimal trichotillomania symptoms) at both time points. Conversely, children assigned to the minimal attention condition did not show improvements in trichotillomania severity, and none were classified as excellent responders. Furthermore, the treatment gains seen in the CBT group were still evident at 6-month follow-up, suggesting a low risk of relapse.

CONCLUSION

A growing body of evidence suggests that CBT is efficacious for the treatment of children and adolescents with trichotillomania and that the risk of relapse after treatment discontinuation may be lower than that reported in previous studies using adult samples. As with adult patients, CBT for children and adolescents with trichotillomania includes core components of rapport building and information gathering, psychoeducation, awareness training using self-monitoring, stimulus control, competing response training, and relapse prevention strategies. Additional interventions such as relaxation training or cognitive restructuring may be applied on an as-needed basis, although they do not replace the core components.

There is a need for much more research on the treatment of pediatric trichotillomania. More randomized trials of CBT are needed, including trials that compare CBT with credible psychotherapy control conditions. In addition, to date, no trials have compared CBT with pharmacotherapy or investigated the addition of pharmacotherapy to CBT in pediatric trichotillomania samples. In adults, CBT generally appears superior to serotonergic antidepressants (Ninan et al. 2000; van Minnen et al. 2003), although the literature on this topic is extremely sparse, and it is not clear whether the same pattern of results would be obtained in children. Given the historical problem of relapse in trichotillomania research, future CBT studies should continue to evaluate this problem carefully, over longer periods of time, making adjustments to the protocol as needed. Finally, as has been done with pediatric obsessive-compulsive disorder (Valderhaug et al. 2007), researchers should conduct effectiveness studies to determine whether the treatment effects seen in research settings can be successfully implemented in nonacademic community mental health settings.

REFERENCES

Azrin NH, Nunn RG: Habit-reversal: a method of eliminating nervous habits and tics. Behav Res Ther 11:619–628, 1973

Beck JS: Cognitive Therapy: Basics and Beyond. New York, Guilford, 1995

Bernstein DA, Borkovec T: Progressive Relaxation Training: A Manual for the Helping Professions. Champaign, IL, Research Press, 1973

Bloch MH, Landeros-Weisenberger A, Dombrowski P, et al: Systematic review: pharmacological and behavioral treatment for trichotillomania. Biol Psychiatry 62:839–846, 2007

Brady RE, Diefenbach GJ, Tolin DF, et al: What works in CBT for trichotillomania: patients' self-report of efficacy. Paper presented at the annual meeting of the Association for Behavioral and Cognitive Therapies, Washington, DC, November 2005

Christenson GA, Ristvedt SL, Mackenzie TB: Identification of trichotillomania cue profiles. Behav Res Ther 31:315–320, 1993

Diefenbach GJ, Tolin DF, Hannan S, et al: Group treatment for trichotillomania: behavior therapy versus supportive therapy. Behav Ther 37:353–363, 2006

Flessner CA, Conelea CA, Woods DW, et al: Styles of pulling in trichotillomania: exploring differences in symptom severity, phenomenology, and functional impact. Behav Res Ther 46:345–357, 2008

Franklin ME, Tolin DF: Treating Trichotillomania: Cognitive Behavior Therapy for Hair Pulling and Related Problems. New York, Springer, 2007

Franklin ME, Tolin DF, Diefenbach GJ: Trichotillomania, in Clinical Manual of Impulse Control Disorders. Edited by Hollander E, Stein DJ. Washington, DC, American Psychiatric Publishing, 2006, pp 149–173

Franklin ME, Cahill SP, Roth Ledley DA, et al: Behavior therapy for pediatric trichotillomania: a randomized controlled trial. Paper presented at the World Congress of Behavioral and Cognitive Therapies, Barcelona, Spain, July 2007

Gluhoski VL: A cognitive approach for treating trichotillomania. J Psychother Pract Res 4:277–285, 1995

Kendall PC: Child and Adolescent Therapy: Cognitive-Behavioral Procedures, 3rd Edition. New York, Guilford, 2006

Lerner J, Franklin ME, Meadows EA, et al: Effectiveness of a cognitive-behavioral treatment program for trichotillomania: an uncontrolled evaluation. Behav Ther 29:157–171, 1998

Mansueto CS: Typography and phenomenology of trichotillomania. Paper presented at the annual meeting of the Association for Advancement of Behavior Therapy, San Francisco, CA, November 1990

Mansueto CS, Stemberger RMT, Thomas AM, et al: Trichotillomania: a comprehensive behavioral model. Clin Psychol Rev 17:567–577, 1997

March JS, Mulle K: OCD in Children and Adolescents: A Cognitive-Behavioral Treatment Manual. New York, Guilford, 1998

Masters JC, Burish TG, Hollon SD, et al: Behavior Therapy: Techniques and Empirical Findings, 3rd Edition. New York, Harcourt Brace Jovanovich, 1987

Mouton SG, Stanley MA: Habit reversal training for trichotillomania: a group approach. Cogn Behav Pract 3:159–182, 1996

Ninan PT, Rothbaum BO, Marsteller FA, et al: A placebo-controlled trial of cognitive-behavioral therapy and clomipramine in trichotillomania. J Clin Psychiatry 61:47–50, 2000

Parks GA, Anderson BK, Marlatt GA: Relapse prevention therapy, in International Handbook of Alcohol Dependence and Problems. Edited by Heather N, Peters TJ, Stockwell T. New York, Wiley, 2001, pp 575–592

Penzel F: The Hair-Pulling Problem: A Complete Guide to Trichotillomania. New York, Oxford University Press, 2003

Stein DJ, Christenson GA, Hollander E (eds): Trichotillomania. Washington, DC, American Psychiatric Press, 1999

Tolin DF, Franklin ME, Diefenbach GJ: Cognitive-behavioral treatment of pediatric trichotillomania: an open trial, in Trichotillomania: Theory and Treatment. Symposium presented at the 31st Congress of the European Association of Behavioral and Cognitive Therapies, Maastricht, The Netherlands, September 2002

Tolin DF, Franklin ME, Diefenbach GJ, et al: Pediatric trichotillomania: descriptive psychopathology and an open trial of cognitive behavioral therapy. Cogn Behav Ther 36:129–144, 2007

Valderhaug R, Larsson B, Gotestam KG, et al: An open clinical trial of cognitive-behaviour therapy in children and adolescents with obsessive-compulsive disorder administered in regular outpatient clinics. Behav Res Ther 45:577–589, 2007

van Minnen A, Hoogduin KA, Keijsers GP, et al: Treatment of trichotillomania with behavioral therapy or fluoxetine. Arch Gen Psychiatry 60:517–522, 2003

Woods DW, Miltenberger RG: Tic Disorders, Trichotillomania, and Other Repetitive Behavior Disorders: Behavioral Approaches to Analysis and Treatment. Norwell, MA, Kluwer Academic Publishers, 2001

Chapter 10

COGNITIVE-BEHAVIORAL THERAPY IN ADULTS

Douglas W. Woods, Ph.D.
Ivar Snorrason, M.A.
Flint M. Espil, M.A.

In this chapter, we discuss cognitive-behavioral therapy (CBT), the most common form of psychotherapy for trichotillomania and chronic skin picking. Reflecting current research trends, coverage in this chapter is weighted toward trichotillomania, but existing research on skin picking is also discussed.

The most common treatments for persons with trichotillomania and skin picking are pharmacotherapy and psychotherapy (Tucker et al. 2011; Woods et al. 2006a). Nevertheless, it is important to note that not all psychotherapies are identical. Different types of therapy are based on different models of understanding mental health issues, and these different models have varying degrees of empirical support. CBT is based on behavioral models of understanding psychiatric problems. Behavioral models have significant research support for understanding the maintenance of various psychiatric problems, including trichotillomania and skin picking. Our purpose in this chapter is to present briefly the behavioral model on which CBT for these disorders is based, describe the core clinical components and structure of CBT, and then review the literature on the efficacy of CBT for trichotillomania and skin picking.

BEHAVIORAL MODEL OF TRICHOTILLOMANIA IN ADULTS

Although behavioral models have focused on understanding the factors maintaining trichotillomania, there is a general belief that the models for trichotillomania also apply to skin picking. Mansueto et al. (1997) presented a comprehensive behavioral model of trichotillomania that proposed functional links between various behavioral, cognitive, and affective variables and trichotillomania (a similar model was proposed by Franklin and Tolin [2007]). This model posited that external (e.g., tools used in pulling, such as tweezers; specific locations, such as bathrooms or bedrooms; or certain activities, such as drawing or reading) and internal (e.g., affective states or cognitions) factors become cues that trigger pulling. In addition, certain consequences of pulling (e.g., pleasurable feelings and reduction in negative states) are believed to maintain the behavior through operant conditioning (i.e., positive and negative reinforcement). Treatments resulting from the model focus on identifying the various triggers and reinforcers for the pulling and developing individual treatment programs to target these functions. In the following subsections, we discuss the various factors believed to maintain and/or exacerbate pulling and picking.

Antecedents Controlling Pulling/Picking

Over time, various stimuli become associated with an urge to pull and eventually become cues to pull or pick. Most people with trichotillomania and skin picking are more likely to pull or pick when in particular settings or during particular activities (Christenson and Mackenzie 1994; Wilhelm et al. 1999). For example, many sufferers are more likely to pull or pick when engaged in sedentary activity (e.g., studying, talking on the telephone, or watching television) and during particular times of the day (e.g., in the evenings). It is also common for people to develop ancillary routines when doing the behavior. For instance, some individuals always use the same implements (e.g., tweezers, mirrors), and others often pull or pick in the same settings (e.g., in the bathroom or bedroom). Various visual (e.g., gray hairs or hairs perceived to be out of place) or tactile (e.g., thick, wiry, or stubbly hair or skin imperfections) stimuli can also trigger the behavior.

A variety of internal states can instigate pulling and picking. Affective states such as tension, anxiety, and boredom can trigger both behaviors (Christenson et al. 1993; Diefenbach et al. 2002, 2008; Neal-Barnett and Stadulis 2006; Snorrason et al. 2010), as can a range of other negative emotions, such as anger, depression, guilt, frustration, and loneliness (Mansueto et al. 1997). Many people with trichotillomania and skin picking report bodily sensations (e.g., general tension, inner pressure) before pulling hair or picking skin (Wetterneck et al. 2005), and some experience an itching sensation prior to the behavior (Arnold et al. 1998; Christenson et al. 1991). In some instances, specific cognitions or thoughts can trigger pulling and picking. For example, patients may have excessive concern about symmetry (e.g., "my eyebrows are uneven") or set beliefs about appearance (e.g., "gray hairs are unacceptable"; "I have to have smooth skin"; Arnold et al. 1998; Mansueto et al. 1997). In addition, a small minority of those with trichotillomania or skin picking will admit to harm-avoidant obsessive thinking in relation to pulling or picking (i.e., engage in the behavior in order to prevent something bad from happening; Arnold et al. 1998; Woods et al. 2006a).

Consequences Controlling Pulling

Many people with trichotillomania and skin picking report gratification and/ or pleasurable feelings during or immediately after the pulling/picking (Diefenbach et al. 2002, 2008; Neal-Barnett and Stadulis 2006; Snorrason et al. 2010; Wilhelm et al. 1999). Similarly, many patients experience reinforcing sensory or tactile stimulation when playing with the hair or the skin, either during or after pulling/picking (e.g., fondling the hair, stroking it with the mouth, rolling the skin between the fingers; Christenson et al. 1991; Rapp et al. 1999; Wilhelm et al. 1999). Additionally, in some people, these behaviors are rewarded through "just right" experiences (e.g., achieving symmetry between eyebrows or smooth skin; Mansueto et al. 1997; Woods et al. 2006a).

Hair pulling and skin picking may also yield negative reinforcers. Many patients report negative emotions (e.g., anxiety, boredom, tension) just before pulling or picking and a significant reduction in these emotions afterwards (Diefenbach et al. 2002, 2008; Neal-Barnett and Stadulis 2006; Snorrason et al. 2010). For some, pulling or picking episodes provide relief from distressing thoughts (e.g., "I have too much to do") or escape from daily existence (e.g., "I go into a trance and forget my troubles for a while"). Ironically, even though hair pulling or skin picking may reduce or eliminate aversive experiences, these behaviors can also intensify certain negative emotions, such as guilt, shame, or general anxiety (e.g., Diefenbach et al. 2002; Woods et al. 2006a). These feelings may in turn trigger later pulling or picking episodes, forming a vicious cycle as the behavior produces the negative states that trigger it (Diefenbach et al. 2002; Mansueto et al. 1997).

Automatic and Focused Pulling

Using the aforementioned controlling factors as a guide, researchers have suggested there may be at least two different styles of hair pulling and skin picking (Christenson and Mackenzie 1994; Walther et al. 2009). *Focused* pulling/picking is performed with full awareness and typically involves pulling or picking in response to internal events such as an urge, negative affect, or specific cognitions. In contrast, *automatic* pulling/picking involves little reflective awareness of the act. Automatic pulling/picking often occurs during sedentary activities (e.g., reading, watching television), and the individual typically does not notice the behavior until afterwards. Only a small minority of people with trichotillomania or skin picking engage exclusively in either focused or automatic pulling/picking; most experience both automatic and focused episodes (du Toit et al. 2001; Flessner et al. 2008; Walther et al. 2009). Nevertheless, many patients will demonstrate a greater tendency for one or the other, which may be important because different styles may respond to different types of intervention. For example, habit reversal training (HRT) and stimulus control strategies (described later) may be especially beneficial for treating automatic pulling/picking, whereas treatment strategies aimed at managing urges, negative affect, and dysfunctional cognitions may be more useful for focused pulling/picking.

Emotion Regulation Mechanisms

Support for the notion that hair pulling and skin picking serve an emotion-regulating function comes from studies examining affective states at different points in the hair-pulling/skin-picking episode (Diefenbach et al. 2002, 2008; Neal-Barnett and Stadulis 2006; Snorrason et al. 2010). As noted earlier, many patients who report negative affective states prior to pulling/picking experience marked reduction in these states after the act, suggesting that the behavior effectively moderates these emotions. Other studies have shown that people with trichotillomania and skin picking often have significantly greater difficulty in managing emotions when compared with healthy control subjects, and experience more severe trichotillomania symptoms as the level of difficulties increases (Shusterman et al. 2009; Snorrason et al. 2010). Taken together, empirical findings suggest that hair pulling and skin picking are effective (albeit maladaptive) emotion regulation strategies and that general difficulties in emotion regulation may underlie the problems.

Other studies have illustrated that the tendency to control private experiences (e.g., unwanted cognitions or emotions) is more central to these problems than the experience of the emotion per se. Evidence for this comes from two areas. First, it has been found that a general tendency to avoid or escape aversive private experiences (i.e., experiential avoidance) is associated with greater hair-pulling and skin-picking severity (Begotka et al. 2004; Flessner and Woods 2006; Norberg et al. 2007). Second, studies show that experiential avoidance mediates the relation between trichotillomania severity and both unpleasant emotions (Wetterneck and Woods 2007) and dysfunctional cognitions (Norberg et al. 2007). Similarly, Flessner and Woods (2006) reported that experiential avoidance mediates the relation between negative affect and skin-picking severity. Although preliminary, these findings indicate that the more the individual seeks to escape from or avoid unwanted private experiences, the more likely he or she is to pull hair or pick skin in response to unpleasant thoughts or emotions.

COGNITIVE-BEHAVIORAL THERAPY FOR TRICHOTILLOMANIA AND SKIN PICKING

Based on the aforementioned behavioral model, CBT seeks to modify the various antecedents and consequences maintaining pulling/picking, with the understanding that consistent application of cognitive-behavioral techniques will result in relatively permanent changes to brain functioning. In nearly all forms of CBT for trichotillomania and skin picking, the core elements of treatment can roughly be divided into two groups—one set of techniques designed to address variables exacerbating and maintaining automatic pulling and another set for focused pulling. Although these are described separately, CBT typically involves all of the techniques; however, some may be emphasized more than others depending on the age of the client and/or the particular function hair pulling seems to serve. CBT interventions targeting the different functions are described in the following section.

Strategies for Addressing Automatic Pulling and Picking

Stimulus Control

When teaching a client stimulus control, the therapist should conduct a thorough assessment of the antecedents and consequences related to pulling and picking. The therapist can use the Stimulus Control Assessment Form (Woods and Twohig 2008) to help the client identify situations associated with various levels of pulling and picking. When conducting the assessment, the therapist should rely on the client's verbal report and ask the client to self-monitor his or her pulling/picking on a daily basis. As pulling/picking episodes occur, the client should note where (i.e., settings) and when (i.e., time of day, activities the client may be engaged in) the behavior occurs, what he or she is thinking and feeling before and after pulling/picking, what he or she does with the hair before and after it is pulled, and how emotions and thoughts change after the behavior.

After conducting a detailed assessment of the antecedents, pulling and picking behaviors, and consequences of pulling and picking, the therapist and client can work together to develop interventions to decrease these behaviors. The overall goal of stimulus control is to choose interventions that make pulling and picking more difficult or to provide alternate forms of the positive reinforcement typically produced by these behaviors. Table 10–1 shows common stimulus control interventions for various pulling and picking situations.

Habit Reversal Training

Habit reversal training is another core component in CBT for people with trichotillomania and skin picking. HRT consists of three steps: awareness training, competing response training, and social support.

The first step, *awareness training*, involves describing the pulling or picking, describing preceding sensations and behaviors, and acknowledging pulling/picking (Woods and Twohig 2008). Often, pulling/picking occurs outside of awareness, and patients have not considered the chain of behaviors that ultimately results in damage to hair and skin. To increase the person's awareness, a detailed description of the pulling/picking is needed. The client is asked to provide descriptions of what pulling episodes look like. If the client has difficulty describing these episodes, it may be helpful to have him or her simulate an episode during the session. Descriptions should be highly detailed and include any sensations or behaviors that occur before the pulling or picking. Preceding sensations include signals or warning signs that occur just before the pulling or picking begins. Preceding sensations may be different across clients, but people with trichotillomania and skin picking often describe a vague urge, a tingling sensation on the skin, a feeling of being overwhelmed, or a sense of tension. Preceding behavioral signals might include playing with the hair, rubbing the skin, bringing the hand toward the pulling/picking site, or trying to find the one hair that is "out of place." Clients should work toward identifying two or three warning signs.

After establishing a description of the pulling or picking and its warning signs, the therapist asks the client to identify these behaviors in session. As each pulling/picking episode or warning sign occurs, the client raises a finger in acknowledgment. If the client is uncomfortable pulling or picking in session, he or she may simulate an episode and warning signs in the session, raising a finger as each occurs.

The second step of HRT, *competing response training*, involves teaching the client to engage in a behavior that prevents pulling or picking. This behavior, called a competing response, is done for 1 minute as soon as the client notices he or she is pulling/picking or if any warning signs occur. A commonly used competing response is having clients fold their arms or place their arms at their sides and gently clench their fists. Whatever the therapist and client decide to use for a competing response, it is important that the action be 1) physically incompatible with the pulling or picking behavior, 2) usable in almost any situation, 3) unnoticeable to others, and 4) acceptable to the client (Woods and Twohig 2008).

TABLE 10–1.   **Stimulus control interventions**

Sample situation	Possible intervention
Bedtime	Only go to bed when tired; if unable to fall asleep after 5 minutes, get up and return to bed when tired.
In front of mirror	Remove mirrors, limit time in front of mirror.
Reading	Hold another object such as a pencil in free hand or hold a book with both hands.
Bathroom	Use a timer to limit time in bathroom, dim lights to decrease visibility, remove mirrors from bathroom.
Driving	Keep both hands on the wheel, remove sharp objects and other tools used for picking and pulling from the vehicle.
Using sharp objects and tools	Remove all sharp objects (pins, needles, tweezers) from house and handbags.
Playing with pulled hair	Provide alternative stimuli such as strings or soft, furry objects to manipulate in high-risk times.
Rubbing pulled hair between fingers	Wear gloves or finger covers during high-risk times to attenuate sensation from fingers.

After deciding on an appropriate competing response, the therapist should demonstrate the exercise for the client. The competing response should be used when the client pulls/picks (or experiences warning signs) and should be held for 1 minute. If the urge returns at the end of 1 minute, the client should repeat the competing response for an additional minute. After the therapist demonstrates the competing response, the client practices the correct use of the competing response in session.

The final component of HRT involves enlisting a *social support* person, such as a friend, relative, or romantic partner, who is asked to point out the client's behavior to help him or her become more aware and gently remind him or her to practice the competing response.

Strategies for Treating Focused Pulling and Picking

Emotion Regulation Issues

In addition to stimulus control and HRT, there are a number of direct and indirect change strategies to help clients reduce pulling and picking and cope with difficulties in emotion regulation. Direct change strategies include relaxation training and cognitive restructuring. Because negative emotions such as stress can increase the risk of pulling (Christenson et al. 1993), progressive muscle relaxation (PMR) training can be used to help clients relieve tension that may put them at greater risk. Although PMR was developed to treat clients with anxiety disorders (Goldfried and Davison 1994), it may be useful for some people with trichotillomania or skin picking. In PMR, the therapist instructs the client to tense and relax several muscle groups throughout the body in order to increase the client's awareness of muscle tension. When PMR is included with HRT and stimulus control in a treatment package for trichotillomania, clients may report PMR as less helpful compared with the other components of treatment (Franklin and Tolin 2007), but clients who also have elevated symptoms of anxiety report PMR to be more helpful and use it more often (Brady et al. 2005).

Another direct change strategy to help clients with emotion regulation issues is cognitive restructuring. *Cognitive restructuring* is the process of evaluating, challenging, and changing maladaptive core beliefs that often perpetuate a problem (Beck 1995). Given that many people may pull or pick to reduce negative/irrational thoughts or emotions (Woods et al. 2006b), identifying and altering cognitive precursors to pulling or picking may be important in treatment. If negative or irrational thoughts precede pulling and picking, the restructuring techniques might be used to identify and alter these thoughts in order to reduce these episodes. Likewise, if negative thoughts contribute to anxiety or depression and if pulling or picking manages such feelings, then altering the negative thoughts may decrease negative emotions, thereby reducing pulling/picking.

Indirect change strategies used to help clients address emotion regulation issues include acceptance-based strategies and mindfulness. Using acceptance-based strategies, the therapist teaches the client to accept, rather than to avoid or control, urges to pull or pick. This strategy is borrowed from acceptance and commitment therapy (ACT; Hayes et al. 1999), which emphasizes the acceptance of negative private events (i.e., thoughts, emotions, images, urges) while engaging in behavior consistent with personal values. When teaching acceptance, the therapist should be clear about the *target* of acceptance. Although the client may be able to reduce pulling or picking through HRT and stimulus control, he or she may continue to experience urges and the negative emotions that precipitate pulling and picking. Acceptance involves experiencing the urges, cognitions, and other emotional experiences for what they are and letting them pass without acting on them. *Acceptance* in this case does not mean resignation to a lifetime of pulling or picking.

Acceptance involves a component of mindfulness, a technique that teaches patients to relate to experiences in a way that minimizes the impact of aversive events (Germer et al. 2005). Mindfulness can help clients experience urges, negative thoughts, and negative emotions (e.g., depression, anxiety, frustration) as they occur in the present moment. Clients continue to be mindful of negative thoughts and emotions until they pass. Because attempts to remove disturbing private events often intensify such events, clients learn to let negative thoughts and emotions come and go (Germer et al. 2005). Instead of trying to avoid urges, clients can use mindfulness to recognize an urge is present until it passes. Although mindfulness has not been empirically validated as a treatment for trichotillomania or skin picking, it has been effective as part of an acceptance-based treatment component (Woods and Twohig 2008) and with dialectical behavior therapy for pulling and picking (DBT; Keuthen et al. 2010).

Clinical Considerations

Pulling and Picking Styles

When treating clients with trichotillomania or skin picking, the therapist may emphazsize different treatment components depending on the predominant style of pulling/picking (i.e., focused vs. automatic). To aid in assessing the relative strength of focused and automatic styles, the therapist may find it useful to use one of three scales. On the Milwaukee Inventory for Subtypes of Trichotillomania (MIST; Flessner et al. 2007b), clients rate the degree to which each statement fits with their own pulling behavior. Total scores are calculated for automatic pulling and focused pulling. Clients under the age of 18 should use the version for children (MIST-C; Flessner et al. 2007a), and clients 18 and over should be given the version for adults (MIST-A; Flessner et al. 2007b). If the client endorses more focused pulling, greater emphasis on interventions such as cognitive restructuring and acceptance of urges may be necessary. If the client endorses more automatic pulling, stimulus control and awareness training may be especially important. Therapists should follow the same detailed assessment procedures when evaluating skin picking. The Milwaukee Inventory for the Dimensions of Adult Skin Picking (MIDAS; Walther et al. 2009) may be helpful for this purpose.

Therapists should be careful not to assume that all clients are motivated to change. Although trichotillomania/skin picking may cause significant distress and impairment, clients often report enjoying the act itself or learn to live with it despite the complications. In cases in which the client is not ready or willing to change, trying to rush into or force treatment not only will lessen the chance of success but also may deter clients from seeking treatment when they are eventually ready to change.

When motivational concerns are present, it may be useful to add strategies to enhance motivation, such as those used in motivational interviewing (Miller and Rollnick 2002). A variety of techniques outlined by Miller and Rollnick (2002), such as expressing empathy, helping clients see the discrepancy between where they are now and where they would be if they were to stop pulling or picking, avoiding argumentation, rolling with resistance from clients, and supporting any efforts to make changes, may be helpful. Some CBTs for trichotillomania include a motivational enhancement component using these techniques (Franklin and Tolin 2007).

Psychoeducation/Support

Clients may be unaware of how common pulling and picking are in the general population and are often surprised to learn that others engage in many of the same behaviors (e.g., trying to find the perfect hair, picking at skin until it bleeds, chewing or swallowing hair). Providing the client with knowledge of the disorder and the understanding that he or she is not alone can be very empowering. The therapist can also educate those close to the client about the nature, course, and treatment of the problem and take the opportunity to explore and address any family problems that may be present due to previous family interactions surrounding the disorder. Therapists can review the importance of reinforcing non-pulling/picking behaviors and avoiding the punishing style of family interactions that can happen when pulling or picking occurs. Sometimes, a reward system is developed to reinforce utilization of treatment techniques (Franklin and Tolin 2007).

EFFICACY OF COGNITIVE-BEHAVIORAL THERAPY FOR TRICHOTILLOMANIA AND CHRONIC SKIN PICKING

Azrin et al. (1980) randomly assigned 34 self-identified hair pullers to either single-session HRT or single-session massed negative practice training. Self-monitoring data obtained 4 weeks after treatment showed the number of hair-pulling episodes decreased more than 90% in the HRT group and slightly more than 50% in the negative practice group. Although promising, this study was limited by the lack of independent outcome measures and failure to establish a diagnosis of trichotillomania.

In a later randomized controlled trial (van Minnen et al. 2003), 40 persons with trichotillomania were assigned to one of three conditions: 1) six biweekly sessions consisting of HRT-like procedures and self-reinforcement, 2) 12-week fluoxetine drug treatment, or 3) 12-week waiting list condition. At posttreatment, 64% of the HRT group showed clinically significant improvement, but only 9% in the fluoxetine group and 20% in the wait-list group met this criterion. The difference between the latter two groups was not significant.

Some authors have examined the efficacy of HRT combined with traditional cognitive interventions. In an uncontrolled trial, Lerner et al. (1998) examined the efficacy of a CBT package consisting of HRT, stimulus control, relaxation training, cognitive restructuring, and relapse prevention methods. At the end of a 9-week treatment phase, 12 out of 14 completers (86%) were classified as treatment responders (i.e., at least a 50% reduction in clinician-rated symptom severity). Ninan et al. (2000) compared the efficacy of a similar CBT package to clomipramine and pill placebo in a randomized controlled trial. According to independent clinician ratings of trichotillomania severity, nine weekly CBT sessions ($n=5$) were more effective than a 9-week clomipramine treatment ($n=6$), which in turn was more effective than a 9-week pill placebo treatment ($n=5$).

The combination of HRT and ACT has also produced promising results. Twohig and Woods (2004) investigated the efficacy of a seven-session acceptance-enhanced behavior therapy (AEBT), which combined HRT with stimulus control and ACT. Patient self-monitoring at posttreatment showed that hair pulling was reduced to a near-zero level in four out of six participants. This treatment package was then developed further and examined in a randomized controlled trial (Woods et al. 2006b) in which trichotillomania patients were assigned to either 10 weekly AEBT sessions ($n=12$) or a 10-week waiting list condition ($n=13$). Self-reported symptom severity on a standardized measure after treatment showed that 66% of the AEBT group demonstrated clinically significant improvement, compared with only 8% of subjects in the wait-list control group. These findings were corroborated by blinded clinician impairment ratings.

Recently, Keuthen et al. (2010) reported findings from an open, uncontrolled trial in which 10 subjects with trichotillomania received 11 weekly therapy sessions consisting of DBT and HRT. Subjects were also given four maintenance sessions over a 3-month period following treatment. According to independent clinician ratings and participant self-reports, 8 subjects (80%) were considered responders at posttreatment, and all of them maintained their gain through the 3-month maintenance phase.

Finally, Bloch et al. (2007) conducted a meta-analysis of the results from randomized controlled trials comparing HRT-based treatments (Ninan et al. 2000; van Minnen et al. 2003; Woods et al. 2006b) with comparison (i.e., selective serotonin reuptake inhibitor or clomipramine) or control (i.e., wait-list) conditions. Using data from studies relying on blinded assessment of outcome, the authors found that HRT-based treatments were superior to the comparison and control conditions.

The literature on the effectiveness of CBT for skin picking is less robust. However, the few existing studies demonstrate similar findings. Research has shown that HRT alone (Twohig and Woods 2001) and HRT in combination with cognitive therapy (Deckersbach et al. 2002) are effective in reducing skin picking. Also, preliminary evidence suggests that ACT alone (Twohig et al. 2006) or in conjunction with HRT (Flessner et al. 2008) may benefit people with chronic skin picking. Only one randomized controlled trial has examined the efficacy of CBT in treating this disorder. In this study, 25 individuals with skin picking were randomly assigned to either HRT or a wait-list condition (Teng et al. 2006). Results showed that HRT was significantly more effective in reducing skin picking than the wait-list condition. Findings were corroborated with independent ratings of photographs of the damaged areas.

Group Versus Individual Therapy

In addition to being economical and time efficient, a group format can provide social support that may be especially helpful for people with an under-recognized disorder such as trichotillomania (or skin picking). Three studies have tested group-based HRT for trichotillomania. Mouton and Stanley (1996) reported on two separate trials examining the efficacy of six weekly HRT sessions. In the first ($n=3$), all group members achieved substantial reduction in trichotillomania severity at posttreatment according to clinician-rated assessment. In the second trial, four out of five participants gained substantial decreases in clinician-rated pulling severity. Later, Diefenbach et al. (2006) compared the efficacy of HRT group therapy ($n=12$) and a supportive therapy ($n=12$) in a randomized trial. Results showed greater reduction in pulling severity for the HRT group compared with the supportive therapy group. However, only two participants in the HRT group (16.7%) achieved clinically significant change with treatment. This proportion was much smaller than that reported in the study by van Minnen et al. (2003; 64% responders), prompting Diefenbach et al. to conclude that group format may not maximize the potential effects of HRT.

Long-Term Maintenance

Trichotillomania and skin picking are typically chronic problems, and results have been mixed with respect to the durability of treatment gains. The self-identified hair pullers receiving HRT in the Azrin et al. (1980) study generally maintained their gains 22 months after treatment, although only 12 out of 19 subjects were available at follow-up. Woods et al. (2006b) reported that patients receiving AEBT showed maintenance of gains at 3-month follow-up, and Teng et al. (2006) reported that skin-picking subjects responding to HRT generally maintained their gains through 3-month follow-up.

Conversely, other studies have found high relapse rates. In the Lerner et al. (1998) study, 12 of 14 (86%) trichotillomania subjects had clinically significant improvement at posttreatment, but only 4 out of 13 (31%) were still rated clinically improved during long-term follow-up (on average, 3.9 years). Also, treatment gains for the HRT group in the van Minnen et al. (2003) study were reduced by 49% at 3-month follow-up and by 70% at 2-year follow-up (Keijsers et al. 2006). Similarly, studies examining group HRT have reported high relapse rates during 6-month follow-up (Diefenbach et al. 2006; Mouton and Stanley 1996). In summary, studies examining maintenance of treatment gains have reported mixed results.

Predictors of Treatment Response and Long-Term Maintenance

Researchers have tried to identify factors within the patients or the treatment that can predict treatment response or long-term maintenance. Although compliance with CBT procedures has been shown to predict trichotillomania symptom improvement at posttreatment (Woods et al. 2006b), complete abstinence from hair pulling at the end of treatment is associated with good long-term outcome (Diefenbach et al. 2006; Keijsers et al. 2006; Lerner et al. 1998). Some authors have noted pretreatment trichotillomania severity as a predictor of poor maintenance (Lerner et al. 1998), but others have failed to replicate these findings (Keijsers et al. 2006). One study showed that greater reductions in depressive symptoms during therapy were associated with more favorable long-term improvement in trichotillomania symptoms (Keuthen et al. 2000, 2001), but other studies found that lower levels of pretreatment depressive symptoms were related to better long-term outcome (Keijsers et al. 2006; Lerner et al. 1998). Neuroticism, age at trichotillomania onset, and duration of symptoms do not appear to be associated with long-term-gain maintenance (Keijsers et al. 2006; Keuthen et al. 1998; Lerner et al. 1998; Woods et al. 2006b).

Mechanisms of Change

In order to enhance the effectiveness of CBT, it is important to understand the treatment's mechanism of action. In small studies, CBT has been more effective in reducing hair pulling than wait-list conditions (van Minnen et al. 2003; Woods et al. 2006b), supportive therapy (Diefenbach et al. 2006), massed negative practice (Azrin et al. 1980), or pill placebo or drug therapy (Ninan et al. 2000; van Minnen et al. 2003). Based on these findings, it is unlikely that the effect of CBT can be explained entirely by general factors such as passage of time, expectations of recovery, attention from a professional, and/or social support.

From the broader HRT literature, competing response training appears to be a key component (e.g., Miltenberger et al. 1985), but the function of the competing response has not been determined (Miltenberger et al. 1998). The awareness training component may also be uniquely important in establishing the efficacy of HRT. Some authors have found that self-monitoring alone (which presumably enhances awareness) may be sufficient in reducing habit behaviors (e.g., Anthony 1978; Ladouceur 1979). However, very few data are available that can shed light on the mechanisms responsible for the effectiveness of self-monitoring. At least two explanations have been offered (Miltenberger et al. 1998; Woods and Miltenberger 1995). First, making people aware of the habit behavior may simply increase its aversiveness and thus behaviors that stop the habit are reinforced. Second, it might be that self-monitoring contingent on hair pulling produces a mild punishment for the pulling behavior.

From the limited component analysis work, it is believed that the least important part of HRT is the social support component, especially for treatment in adult populations. For example, Flessner et al. (2005) found that HRT without social support was equally effective in reducing nail biting in college students as HRT with the social support component.

Finally, very few empirical data are available that can shed light on the active change mechanism of interventions often applied with HRT, such as ACT, DBT, or CBT techniques. The rationale for using ACT is that experiential avoidance leads people to pull hair or pick skin in response to aversive private experiences. Thus, it is believed that reduction in experiential avoidance will reduce symptoms. Similarly, it is assumed that implementing CBT or DBT helps patients regulate their emotions, which in turn reduces the need to cope with emotions by picking skin or pulling hair. Preliminary evidence supports these notions. Woods et al. (2006b) found that the level of symptom improvement at the end of AEBT was moderately correlated with the change in experiential avoidance. Likewise, Keuthen et al. (2010) reported that reduction in hair-pulling symptoms in patients receiving DBT-enhanced HRT correlated with change in emotion regulation difficulties. These preliminary findings suggest that treatment aimed at helping patients accept or manage negative emotions may reduce hair pulling and possibly skin picking.

REFERENCES

Anthony WZ: Brief intervention in a case of childhood trichotillomania by self-monitoring. J Behav Ther Exp Psychiatry 9:173–175, 1978

Arnold LM, McElroy SL, Mutasim DF, et al: Characteristics of 34 adults with psychogenic excoriation. J Clin Psychiatry 59:509–514, 1998

Azrin NH, Nunn RG, Frantz SE: Treatment of hair pulling (trichotillomania): a comparative study of habit reversal and negative practice training. J Behav Ther Exp Psychiatry 11:13–20, 1980

Beck JS: Cognitive Therapy: Basics and Beyond. New York, Guilford, 1995

Begotka AM, Woods DW, Wetterneck CT: The relationship between experiential avoidance and the severity of trichotillomania in a nonreferred sample. J Behav Ther Exp Psychiatry 35:17–24, 2004

Bloch MH, Landeros-Weisenberger A, Dombrowski P, et al: Systematic review: pharmacological and behavioral treatment for trichotillomania. Biol Psychiatry 62:839–846, 2007

Brady RE, Diefenbach GJ, Tolin DF, et al: What works in CBT for trichotillomania: patients' self-report of efficacy. Paper presented at the annual meeting of the Association for Behavioral and Cognitive Therapies, Washington, DC, November 2005

Christenson GA, Mackenzie TB: Trichotillomania, in Handbook of Prescriptive Treatment for Adults. Edited by Hersen M, Ammerman RT. New York, Plenum, 1994, pp 217–235

Christenson GA, Mackenzie TB, Mitchell JE: Characteristics of 60 adult chronic hair pullers. Am J Psychiatry 148:365–370, 1991

Christenson GA, Ristvedt SL, Mackenzie TB: Identification of trichotillomania cue profiles. Behav Res Ther 31:315–320, 1993

Deckersbach T, Wilhelm S, Keuthen NJ, et al: Cognitive behavior therapy for self-injurious skin picking: a case series. Behav Modif 26:361–377, 2002

Diefenbach GJ, Mouton-Odum S, Stanley MA: Affective correlates of trichotillomania. Behav Res Ther 40:1305–1315, 2002

Diefenbach GJ, Tolin DF, Hannan S, et al: Group treatment for trichotillomania: behavior therapy versus supportive therapy. Behav Ther 37:353–363, 2006

Diefenbach GJ, Tolin DF, Meunier S, et al: Emotion regulation and trichotillomania: a comparison of clinical and nonclinical hair pulling. J Behav Ther Exp Psychiatry 39:32–41, 2008

du Toit PL, van Kradenburg J, Niehaus DJH, et al: Characteristics and phenomenology of hair-pulling: an exploration of subtypes. Compr Psychiatry 42:247–256, 2001

Flessner CA, Woods DW: Phenomenological characteristics, social problems, and the economic impact associated with chronic skin picking. Behav Modif 30:944–963, 2006

Flessner CA, Miltenberger RG, Egemo K, et al: An evaluation of the social support component of simplified habit reversal. Behav Ther 36:35–42, 2005

Flessner CA, Woods DW, Franklin ME, et al: The Milwaukee Inventory for Styles of Trichotillomania—Child Version (MIST-C): initial development and psychometric properties. Behav Modif 31:896–918, 2007a

Flessner CA, Woods DW, Franklin ME, et al: The Milwaukee Inventory for Subtypes of Trichotillomania—Adult Version (MIST-A): development of an instrument for the assessment of "focused" and "automatic" hair pulling. J Psychopathol Behav Assess 30:20–30, 2007b

Flessner CA, Busch AM, Heideman PW, et al: Acceptance-enhanced behavior therapy (AEBT) for trichotillomania and chronic skin picking: exploring the effects of component sequencing. Behav Modif 32:579–594, 2008

Franklin ME, Tolin DF: Treating Trichotillomania: Cognitive-Behavioral Therapy for Hairpulling and Related Problems. New York, Springer, 2007

Germer CK, Siegel RD, Fulton PR (eds): Mindfulness and Psychotherapy. New York, Guilford, 2005

Goldfried MR, Davison GC: Clinical Behavior Therapy. New York, Wiley, 1994

Hayes SC, Strosahl KD, Wilson KG: Acceptance and Commitment Therapy: An Experiential Approach to Behavior Change. New York, Guilford, 1999

Keijsers GP, van Minnen A, Hoogduin CA, et al: Behavioural treatment of trichotillomania: two-year follow-up results. Behav Res Ther 44:359–370, 2006

Keuthen NJ, O'Sullivan RL, Sprich-Buckminster S: Trichotillomania: current issues in conceptualization and treatment. Psychother Psychosom 67:202–213, 2000

Keuthen NJ, Fraim C, Deckersbach T, et al: Longitudinal follow-up of naturalistic treatment outcome in patients with trichotillomania. J Clin Psychiatry 62:101–107, 2001

Keuthen NJ, Rothbaum BO, Welch SS, et al: Pilot trial of dialectical behavior therapy-enhanced habit reversal for trichotillomania. Depress Anxiety 27:953–959, 2010

Ladouceur R: Habit reversal treatment: learning an incompatible response or increasing the subject's awareness? Behav Res Ther 4:313–316, 1979

Lerner J, Franklin ME, Meadows EA, et al: Effectiveness of a cognitive-behavioral treatment program for trichotillomania: an uncontrolled evaluation. Behav Ther 29:157–171, 1998

Mansueto CS, Townsley-Stemberger RM, Thomas A, et al: Trichotillomania: a comprehensive behavioral model. Clin Psychol Rev 17:567–577, 1997

Miller WR, Rollnick S: Motivational Interviewing: Preparing People for Change, 2nd Edition. New York, Guilford, 2002

Miltenberger RG, Fuqua RW, McKinley T: Habit reversal with muscle tics: replication and component analysis. Behav Ther 16:39–50, 1985

Miltenberger RG, Fuqua RW, Woods DW: Applying behavior analysis to clinical problems: review and analysis of habit reversal. J Appl Behav Anal 31:447–469, 1998

Mouton SG, Stanley MA: Habit reversal training for trichotillomania: a group approach. Cogn Behav Pract 3:159–182, 1996

Neal-Barnett AM, Stadulis R: Affective states and racial identity among African American women with trichotillomania. J Natl Med Assoc 98:753–757, 2006

Ninan PT, Rothbaum BO, Marsteller FA, et al: A placebo-controlled trial of cognitive-behavioral therapy and clomipramine in trichotillomania. J Clin Psychiatry 61:47–50, 2000

Norberg MM, Wetterneck CT, Woods DW, et al: Experiential avoidance as a mediator of relationships between cognitions and hair-pulling severity. Behav Modif 31:367–381, 2007

Rapp JT, Miltenberger RG, Galensky TL, et al: A functional analysis of hair pulling. J Appl Behav Anal 32:329–337, 1999

Shusterman A, Feld L, Baer L, et al: Affective regulation in trichotillomania: evidence from a large-scale internet survey. Behav Res Ther 47:637–644, 2009

Snorrason Í, Smári J, Ólafsson RP: Emotion regulation in pathological skin picking: findings from a non–treatment seeking sample. J Behav Ther Exp Psychiatry 41:238–245, 2010

Teng EJ, Woods DW, Twohig MP: Habit reversal as a treatment for chronic skin picking. Behav Modif 30:411–422, 2006

Tucker BTP, Woods DW, Flessner CA, et al: The Skin Picking Impact Project: phenomenology, interference, and treatment utilization of pathological skin picking in a population-based sample. J Anxiety Disord 25:88–95, 2011

Twohig MP, Woods DW: Habit reversal as a treatment for chronic skin picking in typically developing adult male siblings. Behav Modif 34:217–220, 2001

Twohig MP, Woods DW: A preliminary investigation of acceptance and commitment therapy and habit reversal as a treatment for trichotillomania. Behav Ther 35:803–820, 2004

Twohig MP, Hayes SC, Masuda A: A preliminary investigation of acceptance and commitment therapy as a treatment for chronic skin picking. Behav Res Ther 10:1513–1522, 2006

van Minnen A, Hoogduin KA, Keijsers GP, et al: Treatment of trichotillomania with behavioral therapy or fluoxetine. Arch Gen Psychiatry 60:517–522, 2003

Walther MR, Flessner CA, Conelea CA, et al: The Milwaukee Inventory for the Dimensions of Adult Skin Picking (MIDAS): initial development and psychometric properties. J Behav Ther Exp Psychiatry 40:127–135, 2009

Wetterneck CT, Woods DW: A contemporary behavior analytic model of trichotillomania, in Understanding Behavior Disorders: A Contemporary Behavioral Perspective. Edited by Woods DW, Kanter J. Reno, NV, Context Press, 2007, pp 157–180

Wetterneck CT, Woods DW, Flessner CA, et al: Antecedent phenomena associated with trichotillomania: research and treatment implications for an online study. Symposium presented at the Association for Behavior Analysis Conference, Chicago, IL, May 2005

Wilhelm S, Keuthen NJ, Deckersbach T, et al: Self-injurious skin picking: clinical characteristics and comorbidity. J Clin Psychiatry 60:454–459, 1999

Woods DW, Miltenberger RG: Habit reversal: a review of applications and variations. J Behav Ther Exp Psychiatry 26:123–131, 1995

Woods DW, Twohig MP: Trichotillomania: An ACT-Enhanced Behavior Therapy Approach. New York, Oxford University Press, 2008

Woods DW, Flessner CA, Franklin ME, et al: The Trichotillomania Impact Project (TIP): exploring phenomenology, functional impairment, and treatment utilization. J Clin Psychiatry 67:1877–1888, 2006a

Woods DW, Wetterneck CT, Flessner CA: A controlled evaluation of acceptance and commitment therapy plus habit reversal for trichotillomania. Behav Res Ther 44:639–656, 2006b

Chapter 11

ALTERNATIVE TREATMENTS

Jon E. Grant, M.D., M.P.H., J.D.
Samuel R. Chamberlain, M.D., Ph.D.
Brian L. Odlaug, B.A.

As described in previous chapters, treatment trials relating to trichotillomania and other body-focused repetitive behaviors (BFRBs) are relatively few in number. The majority of published trials have considered psychotherapy (notably habit reversal training) and mainstream pharmacological agents such as serotonin reuptake inhibitors (e.g., clomipramine, fluoxetine). This chapter considers other potential interventions for trichotillomania—the so-called alternative treatments—which have received less attention to date. In general terms, selection of treatments for any condition is dependent upon a balance between benefits (clinical efficacy) and costs (side effects, access, monetary costs, time costs). Ideally, aspects of benefits/costs would be evaluated in controlled clinical trials, such as double-blind, randomized, placebo-controlled designs, and in subsequent meta-analyses and systematic reviews. Treatment guidelines for more-studied psychiatric disorders have evaluated studies based on a hierarchy of quality of evidence, ranging from low-level evidence (as seen in case studies/expert opinion and/or uncontrolled studies) through to top-level (from multiple randomized, controlled trials) (e.g., see Bandelow et al. 2008).

As has been seen, even for treatments commonly used for trichotillomania, definitive evidence is often lacking. Unfortunately, this poverty of evidence is even more extreme in the context of alternative treatments, for which in many instances only case reports are available or no peer-reviewed publications exist at all. In our view, alternative treatments should not be used instead of more mainstream treatments; rather, they may have a role in complementing (i.e., may be used concurrently with) more validated treatments. Alternative treatments for trichotillomania were identified by means of examining support Web sites for people with the condition (e.g., the Trichotillomania Learning Center, www.trich.org), searching PubMed or MedLine, and inspecting citation lists of initially identified papers.

AEROBIC EXERCISE

Incorporating aerobic exercise as an adjunct to existing trichotillomania treatment has been proposed as a potentially effective strategy when individuals are still symptomatic despite receiving currently available treatments. In addition to the long-term health benefits of aerobic exercise, research supports the use of aerobic exercise in reducing anxiety and depressive symptoms in clinical and nonclinical populations (Bodin and Martinsen 2004; Broocks et al. 1998; Dunn et al. 2005; Ernst et al. 1998; Martinsen et al. 1989; Petruzzello et al. 1991; Stathopoulou et al. 2006). In fact, one review article found that only 3 of 24 studies examining exercise for anxiety reduction failed to demonstrate anxiety-reducing benefits (Taylor 2000).

Although no data exist for the effects of exercise on trichotillomania, skin picking, or other BFRBs, there is a body of research on its benefits for obsessive-compulsive disorder (OCD), a disorder that has many phenomenological and possibly biological links to trichotillomania and skin picking (e.g., Phillips et al. 2010). One study of 11 subjects with OCD found that a 6-week exercise intervention significantly reduced symptoms (Lancer et al. 2007). A second study of 15 OCD subjects examined 20–40 minutes of aerobic exercise on two or three occasions per week for 12 weeks. Subjects reported small to large reductions in OCD symptoms over the 12-week period (Abrantes et al. 2009).

Individuals with trichotillomania, skin picking, and other BFRBs often report worsening of behaviors related to the intensity of negative mood states and anxiety (Franklin et al. 2008; Mansueto et al. 2007). It is therefore possible that a similar reduction in pulling and picking may occur with exercise. Future studies will be necessary to confirm this hypothesis and to examine how much and for how long exercise may be necessary.

INOSITOL

There is some research supporting the use of inositol in the treatment of compulsive behaviors. Inositol, a glucose isomer and second messenger precursor, regulates numerous cellular functions and has demonstrated efficacy in OCD through mechanisms that remain unclear. Although a small, placebo-controlled study in 13 subjects with OCD found inositol to be more effective than placebo over a 6-week period (Fux et al. 1996), other studies using inositol as an augmentation to an antidepressant in OCD have not demonstrated benefit (Fux et al. 1999; Seedat and Stein 1999), and therefore more research is needed.

In the case of BFRBs, only one formal study reporting the use of inositol has been published. In an open-label study, three women with trichotillomania and skin picking were treated with inositol, and all three improved, with the improvement maintained for the 16 weeks of the study (Seedat et al. 2001). Anecdotal evidence also suggests that inositol may be helpful. Fred Penzel (2003) has used it in his clinic since 1996 and has seen positive results.

With such a dearth of evidence, optimal dosing of inositol is unclear; it has been suggested that anywhere from 2 to 18 grams per day can be effective. Other than a potentially dangerous interaction with lithium, inositol seems to produce few if any side effects (nausea, headache, and diarrhea are possible) (Penzel 2003).

N-ACETYLCYSTEINE

N-Acetylcysteine is an amino acid and antioxidant, and recent research demonstrates that it modulates glutamate within the nucleus accumbens. Glutamatergic dysfunction has been implicated in the pathophysiology of OCD (Chakrabarty et al. 2005), a disorder with both phenomenological and possible neurobiological links to trichotillomania (e.g., Phillips et al. 2010). In addition, clinical reports support the possible efficacy of glutamatergic modulators, such as *N*-acetylcysteine, in the treatment of repetitive or compulsive disorders (Lafleur et al. 2006; Odlaug and Grant 2007). *N*-Acetylcysteine is a hepatoprotective antioxidant that is converted to cystine, a substrate for the glutamate/cystine antiporter. This antiporter allows for the uptake of cystine, causing the reverse transport of glutamate into the extracellular space, which stimulates inhibitory metabotropic glutamate receptors and thereby reduces synaptic release of glutamate (Baker et al. 2003; LaRowe et al. 2006). Restoring extracellular glutamate concentration in the nucleus accumbens appears to block reinstitution of compulsive behaviors.

A double-blind, placebo-controlled study of *N*-acetylcysteine in trichotillomania found that subjects assigned to *N*-acetylcysteine had significantly greater reductions in hair-pulling symptoms compared with those given placebo (Grant et al. 2009). In addition, 56% of the subjects were "much or very much improved" while taking *N*-acetylcysteine (effective dosage range,

1,200–2,400 mg/day), compared with 16% of those given placebo, with significant improvement noted after 9 weeks of the 12-week treatment period. N-Acetylcysteine is available in health food stores, is cheaper than the cost of most insurance copayments, and appears to be well tolerated. Side effects include nausea, indigestion, headache, and abdominal pain, but these have been reported as mild and short term. N-Acetylcysteine should not be used in people with asthma because it may worsen that condition. Many people recommend supplemental zinc, copper, and other trace minerals, as well as taking two to three times the typical amount of vitamin C. These recommendations are based on people taking N-acetylcysteine over an "extended period," and because the scientific literature is unclear as to what that actually means, it is probably best to take N-acetylcysteine with a multivitamin plus vitamin C. People should be cautioned that although N-acetylcysteine is an amino acid and thereby appears safe, people should always ask their doctors before starting the supplement. It is important that people do not mix chemicals, whether they are natural or synthetic or a combination, without a full and complete understanding of the potential interactions. In addition, just because something may be good for you in small doses does not mean that more is better or safe.

A small case series also reported the benefits of N-acetylcysteine in people with skin picking and nail biting (Odlaug and Grant 2007), reporting full remission of symptoms. Current research is examining the use of N-acetylcysteine in pediatric trichotillomania.

ACUPUNCTURE

Acupuncture is an ancient therapeutic technique that has attracted increasing attention from the field of psychiatry (van der Watt et al. 2008). Some research has supported the use of acupuncture for the treatment of anxiety disorders such as OCD (Hollifield et al. 2007). One study examined the addition of acupuncture to medication in treatment-resistant OCD patients (Zhang et al. 2009). The study compared 12 sessions of acupuncture with a wait list in 19 subjects with OCD and found that OCD symptoms showed greater improvement in those receiving acupuncture. The authors suggested that the mechanism of action is enhanced serotonergic activity and/or enhanced endorphin release in the hypothalamus and limbic regions (Zhang et al. 2009). Studies of acupuncture in individuals with BFRBs, however, are lacking.

HYPNOSIS

Hypnosis has a long and colorful history dating from Mesmer's magnetic treatments of 1774 to its use in combat neurosis after World War I. As such, it is a complex, poorly understood phenomenon (Robiner et al. 1999). Multiple definitions of hypnosis have been proposed, and some have characterized hypnosis not as a treatment but as a conduit through which treatments (e.g., cognitive-behavioral therapy) are delivered. Although the mechanisms of symptom reduction are poorly understood, case reports have suggested that hypnosis may be beneficial for some individuals with BFRBs (Robiner et al. 1999).

There are many case reports regarding the use of hypnosis in the treatment of BFRBs, many of which were conducted in children rather than in adults (Arone di Bertolino and Nanni 1980; Barabasz 1987; Bornstein et al. 1980; Cohen et al. 1999; de L Horne 1977; Fabbri and Dy 1974; Galski 1981; Gardner 1978; Gruenewald 1965; Hall and McGill 1986; Hynes 1982; Iglesias 2003; Rowen 1981; Thomson 2002; Zalsman et al. 2001). The goals of hypnosis for these behaviors have differed across case reports. Some approaches have focused on increasing awareness and control over the behaviors, whereas others have targeted reduction in anxiety or tried to increase pain sensitivity (e.g., see Barabasz 1987; Fabbri and Dy 1974; Galski 1981; Hall and McGill 1986; Hynes 1982).

The case reports and series have involved only small numbers of subjects, and no controlled studies have been performed. In addition, hypnosis was often enhanced by other techniques (e.g., restricted environmental stimulation technique, behavioral therapy, group therapy), and the number of hypnotic sessions ranged from 1 to 10. The case reports included follow-up periods of up to 12–18 months and generally demonstrated that most subjects improved and that subjects had moderate to large benefits (e.g., Barabasz 1987; Galski 1981; Kohen 1996; Laser 1990). Although some of the case series include reports of subjects who did not improve (Barabasz 1987; Kohen 1996), without controlled studies it is not possible to characterize the chance of improvement using hypnosis or the relative efficacy or otherwise of this approach.

COSMETIC TECHNIQUES

A variety of techniques have been used by people with trichotillomania in an effort to prevent the hair-pulling habit and to mask or hide the resulting bald patches. The noticeable hair loss integral to trichotillomania has profound deleterious effects on quality of life and social function, often leading to problems with anxiety and depression. Therefore, techniques for masking hair loss are potentially very valuable. It has been documented that many people with trichotillomania use physical items such as hair bands, hats, or wigs in an effort to block pulling behavior (by providing a physical barrier or distraction) and to hide the patches. The utility of these approaches has not been studied in formal trials. However, such methods are generally relatively inexpensive with low risk to the sufferer. More involved and expensive techniques have been developed by several commercial hair studios, which use hair extensions (or even hair replacement) in a variety of hair loss contexts, including trichotillomania, alopecia, and hair loss from chemotherapy/radiotherapy. Although results from such systems appear alluring, there is often considerable cost to the individual; therefore, before recommendations as to their usefulness are made (or before such systems are recognized as formal healthcare treatments), appropriately controlled clinical trials are to be encouraged.

BIOFEEDBACK

Biofeedback refers to the use of various measures to help individuals monitor and alter their physiological status. Examples of biofeedback measures include galvanic skin responses, electromyography, and electroencephalography (Shenefelt 2003). According to some practitioners, biofeedback can allow patients to reduce overall stress levels and to discover alternative ways of relieving stress in order to replace ingrained habits such as BFRBs. For example, muscle feedback can be given from the face, forehead, and neck areas: the focus of patients' attention can thus be shifted away from bad habits onto the replacement "habit" of being preoccupied with reducing muscle tension. Similarly, feedback using abdomen sensors (related to breathing), temperature, and galvanic skin responses can be provided in order to train patients to recognize and therefore reduce tension and arousal.

   Biofeedback is rarely examined in clinical trials, and there have been no published reports of using this technique for BRFBs. There are, however, several case reports suggesting the value of biofeedback in reducing tics, which bear some phenomenological similarities to BFRBs such as hair pulling (Nagai et al. 2009; Tansey 1986).

MEDITATION AND YOGA

Methods capable of reducing anxiety or arousal, besides biofeedback, may also have a role to play in the treatment of BFRBs. There have been no case studies or controlled trials examining the utility of meditation/yoga in moderating trichotillomania, skin picking, or nail-biting symptomatology. In a study conducted in OCD patients, those receiving meditation treatment ($n=8$) showed significant benefits in terms of mindfulness, OCD symptoms, letting go, and thought-action fusion as compared with a wait-list control group ($n=9$)

(Hanstede et al. 2008). Meditation comprised eight group meetings, which taught breathing techniques, body scan, and mindful daily living. Elsewhere, in a controlled trial, patients with OCD were randomly assigned to treatment with either yoga-meditation ($n=11$) or relaxation response plus mindfulness meditation techniques ($n=10$) for 3 months initially (Shannahoff-Khalsa et al. 1999). In an intent-to-treat analysis, significant symptom improvement was found in the former but not in the latter group, suggesting that yoga-meditation can be useful in the treatment of OCD. At 3 months, all subjects were merged to receive yoga-meditation for an additional 12 months; the group showed significant improvements across multiple measures of disease severity.

The pilot studies outlined here suggest that at least some forms of meditation/yoga may be useful in OCD (and therefore, potentially, grooming habits), and there are reasons to believe that such techniques can modulate brain circuitry implicated in the manifestation of trichotillomania as well. Magnetic resonance and diffusion tensor imaging have identified structural abnormalities in emotional processing regions (e.g., amygdala, hippocampus) and their interconnecting white matter tracts in people with trichotillomania (Chamberlain et al. 2008, 2010). Using functional magnetic resonance imaging in conjunction with a thermal pain paradigm, researchers showed that practitioners of (Zen) meditation versus control subjects exhibited reduced activity in neural regions, including the amygdala and hippocampus, during pain (Grant et al. 2011). Elsewhere, it was reported using structural magnetic resonance imaging that meditators showed larger volumes in the hippocampus and orbitofrontal cortex, both of which have been heavily implicated in emotional regulation (Luders et al. 2009). These findings suggest that meditation can influence the structure and function of emotional processing regions also implicated in the pathophysiology of trichotillomania.

CAUTIONS AND RECOMMENDATIONS

In summary, there is evidence from a double-blind, randomized, placebo-controlled trial to support the utility of the amino acid *N*-acetylcysteine in the treatment of trichotillomania, and there are unpublished data and case series to suggest it may be useful for other BFRBs as well. *N*-Acetylcysteine appears to be generally well tolerated, although it should be used under medical supervision and avoided in people with asthma. Expert opinion supports the use of inositol under medical supervision, although it should be avoided in people taking lithium. Several interventions are noteworthy for being low risk and inexpensive and are worth exploring where patients feel they may be useful: aerobic exercise in people without medical conditions (where medical conditions exist, patients should seek physician guidance first) and certain cosmetic interventions (e.g., hair bands, hats, makeup). There is evidence from multiple case reports that hypnotherapy, especially when used as a conduit for other interventions (e.g., psychotherapy), can be useful; however, there have been no controlled trials, and such treatments may be costly. In some people, hair pulling may be driven by hyperarousal and anxiety states (Stein et al. 2006). As such, meditation, prayer, and yoga (which are potentially anxiolytic and reduce arousal) could be useful to some people at relatively low cost and risk. Dietary changes and herbal remedies, although suggested by some, are not supported by available data and involve potential risk. It is worth bearing in mind that trustworthy support Web sites and books represent an important part of the therapeutic process for many patients. In all, we urge caution in the use of alternative treatments that involve undue risk and cost, in the absence of objective scrutiny as to their relative benefits.

REFERENCES

Abrantes AM, Strong DR, Cohn A, et al: Acute changes in obsessions and compulsions following moderate-intensity aerobic exercise among patients with obsessive-compulsive disorder. J Anxiety Disord 23:923–927, 2009

Arone di Bertolino R, Nanni G: Treatment of onychophagia [in Italian]. Minerva Med 71:1269–1272, 1980

Baker DA, McFarland K, Lake RW, et al: N-Acetyl cysteine–induced blockade of cocaine-induced reinstatement. Ann NY Acad Sci 1003:349–351, 2003

Bandelow B, Zohar J, Hollander E, et al: World Federation of Societies of Biological Psychiatry (WFSBP) guidelines for the pharmacological treatment of anxiety, obsessive-compulsive and post-traumatic stress disorders—first revision. World J Biol Psychiatry 9:248–312, 2008

Barabasz M: Trichotillomania: a new treatment. Int J Clin Exp Hypn 35:146–154, 1987

Bodin T, Martinsen EW: Mood and self-efficacy during acute exercise in clinical depression: a randomized, controlled study. J Sport Exerc Psychol 26:623–633, 2004

Bornstein PH, Rychtarik RG, McFall ME, et al: Hypnobehavioral treatment of chronic nailbiting: a multiple baseline analysis. Int J Clin Exp Hypn 28:208–217, 1980

Broocks A, Badelow B, Pekrun G, et al: Comparison of aerobic exercise, clomipramine, and placebo in the treatment of panic disorder. Am J Psychiatry 155:603–609, 1998

Chakrabarty K, Bhattacharyya S, Christopher R, et al: Glutamatergic dysfunction in OCD. Neuropsychopharmacology 30:1735–1740, 2005

Chamberlain SR, Menzies LA, Fineberg NA, et al: Grey matter abnormalities in trichotillomania: morphometric magnetic resonance imaging study. Br J Psychiatry 193:216–221, 2008

Chamberlain SR, Hampshire A, Menzies LA, et al: Reduced brain white matter integrity in trichotillomania: a diffusion tensor imaging study. Arch Gen Psychiatry 67:965–971, 2010

Cohen HA, Barzilai A, Lahat E: Hypnotherapy: an effective treatment modality for trichotillomania. Acta Paediatr Scand 88:407–410, 1999

de L Horne DJ: Behaviour therapy for trichotillomania. Behav Res Ther 15:192–196, 1977

Dunn AL, Trivedi MH, Kampert JB, et al: Exercise treatment for depression: efficacy and dose response. Am J Prev Med 28:1–8, 2005

Ernst E, Rand JI, Stevinson C: Complementary therapies for depression: an overview. Arch Gen Psychiatry 55:1026–1032, 1998

Fabbri R Jr, Dy AJ: Hypnotic treatment of trichotillomania: two cases. Int J Clin Exp Hypn 22:210–215, 1974

Franklin ME, Flessner CA, Woods DW, et al: The Child and Adolescent Trichotillomania Impact Project: descriptive psychopathology, comorbidity, functional impairment, and treatment utilization. J Dev Behav Pediatr 29:493–500, 2008

Fux M, Levine J, Aviv A, et al: Inositol treatment of obsessive-compulsive disorder. Am J Psychiatry 153:1219–1221, 1996

Fux M, Benjamin J, Belmaker RH: Inositol versus placebo augmentation of serotonin reuptake inhibitors in the treatment of obsessive-compulsive disorder: a double-blind cross-over study. Int J Neuropsychopharmacol 2:193–195, 1999

Galski TJ: The adjunctive use of hypnosis in the treatment of trichotillomania: a case report. Am J Clin Hypn 23:198–201, 1981

Gardner GG: Hypnotherapy in the management of childhood habit disorders. J Pediatr 92:838–840, 1978

Grant JA, Courtemanche J, Rainville P: A non-elaborative mental stance and decoupling of executive and pain-related cortices predicts low pain sensitivity in Zen meditators. Pain 152:150–156, 2011

Grant JE, Odlaug BL, Kim SW: N-Acetylcysteine, a glutamate modulator, in the treatment of trichotillomania: a double-blind, placebo-controlled study. Arch Gen Psychiatry 66:756–763, 2009

Gruenewald D: Hypnotherapy in a case of adult nailbiting. Int J Clin Exp Hypn 13:209–219, 1965

Hall JR, McGill JC: Hypnobehavioral treatment of self-destructive behavior: trichotillomania and bulimia in the same patient. Am J Clin Hypn 29:39–46, 1986

Hanstede M, Gidron Y, Nyklícek I: The effects of a mindfulness intervention on obsessive-compulsive symptoms in a non-clinical student population. J Nerv Ment Dis 196:776–779, 2008

Hollifield M, Sinclair-Lian N, Warner TD, et al: Acupuncture for posttraumatic stress disorder: a randomized controlled pilot trial. J Nerv Ment Dis 195:504–513, 2007

Hynes JV: Hypnotic treatment of five adult cases of trichotillomania. Australian Journal of Clinical and Experimental Hypnosis 10:109–116, 1982

Iglesias A: Hypnosis as a vehicle for choice and self-agency in the treatment of children with trichotillomania. Am J Clin Hypn 46:129–137, 2003

Kohen DP: Hypnotherapeutic management of pediatric and adolescent trichotillomania. J Dev Behav Pediatr 17:328–334, 1996

Lafleur DL, Pittenger C, Kelmendi B, et al: N-Acetylcysteine augmentation in serotonin reuptake inhibitor refractory obsessive-compulsive disorder. Psychopharmacology (Berl) 184:254–256, 2006

Lancer R, Motta R, Lancer D: The effect of aerobic exercise on obsessive-compulsive disorder, anxiety, and depression: a preliminary investigation. Behavior Therapist 30:53–62, 2007

LaRowe SD, Mardikian P, Malcolm R, et al: Safety and tolerability of N-acetylcysteine in cocaine-dependent individuals. Am J Addict 15:105–110, 2006

Laser E: Tight squeeze: an Adlerian hypnotherapy of a case of trichotillomania. Individual Psychology Journal of Adlerian Theory, Research and Practice 46:490–497, 1990

Luders E, Toga AW, Lepore N, et al: The underlying anatomical correlates of long-term meditation: larger hippocampal and frontal volumes of gray matter. Neuroimage 45:672–678, 2009

Mansueto CS, Thomas AM, Brice AL: Hair pulling and its affective correlates in an African-American university sample. J Anxiety Disord 21:590–599, 2007

Martinsen EW, Hoffart A, Solberg O: Comparing aerobic with nonaerobic forms of exercise in the treatment of clinical depression: a randomized trial. Compr Psychiatry 30:324–331, 1989

Nagai Y, Cavanna A, Critchley HD: Influence of sympathetic autonomic arousal on tics: implications for a therapeutic behavioral intervention for Tourette syndrome. J Psychosom Res 67:599–605, 2009

Odlaug BL, Grant JE: N-Acetyl cysteine in the treatment of grooming disorders. J Clin Psychopharmacol 27:227–229, 2007

Penzel F: The Hair-Pulling Problem: A Complete Guide to Trichotillomania. New York, Oxford University Press, 2003

Petruzzello SJ, Landers DM, Hatfield BD, et al: A meta-analysis on the anxiety-reducing effects of acute and chronic exercise: outcomes and mechanisms. Sports Med 11:143–182, 1991

Phillips KA, Stein DJ, Rauch SL, et al: Should an obsessive-compulsive spectrum grouping of disorders be included in DSM-V? Depress Anxiety 27:528–555, 2010

Robiner WN, Edwards PE, Christenson GA: Hypnosis in the treatment of trichotillomania, in Trichotillomania. Edited by Stein DJ, Christenson GA, Hollander E. Washington, DC, American Psychiatric Press, 1999, pp 167–199

Rowen R: Hypnotic age regression in the treatment of a self-destructive habit: trichotillomania. Am J Clin Hypn 23:195–197, 1981

Seedat S, Stein DJ: Inositol augmentation of serotonin reuptake inhibitors in treatment-refractory obsessive-compulsive disorder: an open trial. Int Clin Psychopharmacol 14:353–356, 1999. Erratum in Int Clin Psychopharmacol 15:244, 2000

Seedat S, Stein DJ, Harvey BH: Inositol in the treatment of trichotillomania and compulsive skin picking. J Clin Psychiatry 62:60–61, 2001

Shannahoff-Khalsa DS, Ray LE, Levine S, et al: Randomized controlled trial of yogic meditation techniques for patients with obsessive-compulsive disorder. CNS Spectr 4:34–47, 1999

Shenefelt PD: Biofeedback, cognitive-behavioral methods, and hypnosis in dermatology: is it all in your mind? Dermatol Ther 16:114–122, 2003

Stathopoulou GM, Powers MB, Berry AC, et al: Exercise interventions for mental health: a quantitative and qualitative review. Clinical Psychology Science and Practice 13:179–191, 2006

Stein DJ, Chamberlain SR, Fineberg N: An A-B-C model of habit disorders: hair-pulling, skin-picking, and other stereotypic conditions. CNS Spectr 11:824–827, 2006

Tansey MA: A simple and a complex tic (Gilles de la Tourette's syndrome): their response to EEG sensorimotor rhythm biofeedback training. Int J Psychophysiol 4:91–97, 1986

Taylor AH: Physical activity, anxiety, and stress, in Physical Activity and Psychological Well-Being. Edited by Biddle SJH, Fox KR, Boutcher SH. New York, Routledge, 2000, pp 10–45

Thomson L: Hypnosis for habit disorders: helping children help themselves. Adv Nurse Pract 10:59–62, 2002

van der Watt G, Laugharne J, Janca A: Complementary and alternative medicine in the treatment of anxiety and depression. Curr Opin Psychiatry 21:37–42, 2008

Zalsman G, Hermesh H, Sever J: Hypnotherapy in adolescents with trichotillomania: three cases. Am J Clin Hypn 44:63–68, 2001

Zhang LL, Zhang G, Zhang LP: Prof. Zhang Zhi-jun's experience in the combined treatment with acupuncture and Chinese herbs: a report of 3 illustrative cases. J Tradit Chin Med 29:279–282, 2009

Chapter 12

PHARMACOTHERAPY

Samuel R. Chamberlain, M.D., Ph.D.

Naomi A. Fineberg, M.B.B.S., M.R.C.Psych.

Brian L. Odlaug, B.A.

Trichotillomania, pathological skin picking (PSP), and pathological nail biting (onychophagia) are under-researched yet debilitating conditions that overlap with one another in terms of phenomenology and comorbid expression (Bohne et al. 2005; Odlaug and Grant 2008; Stein et al. 2006). Although trichotillomania is recognized in DSM-IV-TR (American Psychiatric Association 2000), PSP and onychophagia are not yet explicitly included, although they may be in future versions of the manual. All three disorders are characterized by repetitive grooming behaviors that are difficult to suppress and often somewhat stereotypical. As such, they may relate to stereotypic movement disorder (DSM-IV-TR 307.3), which is characterized by non-functional and seemingly driven self-injurious behaviors (e.g., hand waving, rocking, playing with hands, twirling objects, and head banging). However, in contrast to stereotypic movement disorder, trichotillomania, PSP, and onychophagia are not typically associated with mental retardation.

In milder forms, hair pulling, picking at one's skin, and nail biting are commonplace behaviors of negligible impact. However, manifested in extreme forms, these habits spiral out of control; induce extreme distress and disability; substantially interfere with social, work, and family life; and trigger comorbidities such as major depression. Relatively little hard evidence exists regarding the population-wide prevalence and epidemiology of these conditions (studies are reviewed fully in Chapter 1, "Trichotillomania: Epidemiology and Clinical Characteristics"; Chapter 2, "Pathological Skin Picking"; and Chapter 3,

"Habitual Stereotypic Movements: A Descriptive Analysis of Four Common Types"). The available surveys suggest lifetime prevalence rates of approximately 0.5%–3.5% for trichotillomania (Christenson et al. 1991b; Franklin et al. 2008; King et al. 1995) and 0.2%–5.4% for PSP (Hayes et al. 2009; Keuthen et al. 2010). The lifetime prevalence rate for onychophagia is not yet established but is thought to be similar to that of PSP (i.e., up to 1.5%) (Bohne et al. 2005). Trichotillomania and PSP share many clinical characteristic similarities as well. Each has a similar gender distribution in the general population, with a high preponderance of females (93.2% and 87.1%–94.1%, respectively) (Arnold et al. 1998; Grant et al. 2010; Wilhelm et al. 1999; Woods et al. 2006), although recent research suggests that a higher proportion of males may have problems with hair pulling (Odlaug and Grant 2010).

Several conceptualizations of trichotillomania, PSP, and onychophagia have been suggested in the literature, and these are not mutually exclusive. In addition to these disorders being viewed as characterized by pathological grooming, they also can be considered body-focused repetitive behaviors (Stein et al. 2007, 2008) or obsessive-compulsive spectrum disorders (Hollander et al. 2007; Swedo and Leonard 1992). The latter stance holds that these disorders bear a relationship with obsessive-compulsive disorder (OCD): along with OCD, they are associated with repetitive behaviors that are difficult to suppress and are likely to be associated, to some extent, with overlapping frontostriatal dysfunction. The concept that these disorders are nosologically related derives some support from the fact that they frequently co-occur within and between each other. For example, the rate of co-occurring OCD has been shown to be significantly higher in individuals with PSP (6%–52%) than in community samples (1%–3%) (Arnold et al. 1998; Simeon et al. 1997; Wilhelm et al. 1999). Similarly, the rate of PSP among individuals with OCD has also been high (8.9%–24.0%) (Cullen et al. 2001; Grant et al. 2006). Furthermore, rates of co-occurring lifetime trichotillomania have been found in 38.3% of a sample of 60 PSP patients (Odlaug and Grant 2007), and research has also indicated high rates of PSP in the first-degree relatives of those with PSP (30.3%–45%) (Odlaug and Grant 2008). Neurobiological data regarding trichotillomania, PSP, and onychophagia are considered later in this chapter.

In contrast to other putatively related disorders such as OCD (Fineberg and Gale 2005), relatively few studies have been undertaken to evaluate, in an objective fashion, the effects of pharmacotherapies on grooming disorders (Chamberlain et al. 2009b). In the current chapter, we review the available clinical trials and case studies, which were identified via PubMed searches and scanning of identified articles' reference lists. Because psychological treatments for these conditions are considered elsewhere (Chapter 9, "Cognitive-Behavioral Therapy for Pediatric Trichotillomania," and Chapter 10, "Cognitive-Behavioral Therapy in Adults"), here we discuss only those therapeutic trials that have also included a pharmacological treatment arm. Blinded and open-label trials are described in detail, and case reports of particular pharmacotherapies are briefly outlined. After reviewing the individual studies, we attempt to draw conclusions for the clinician as to the "strength of evidence" supporting each treatment strategy, based upon the relatively exacting categories of evidence and recommendation grades proposed by Bandelow et al. (2008) (see Table 12–1 later in this chapter). This guideline, built on earlier work by Eccles and Mason (2001), importantly distinguishes categories of evidence (based on efficacy alone) from recommendation grades (which take into account efficacy and any potential advantages/disadvantages of particular drugs—e.g., relating to side effects and interactions).

TRICHOTILLOMANIA

Double-Blind Trials

Randomized, double-blind, controlled trials of small size have been performed in trichotillomania. The earliest trials examined serotonin reuptake inhibitors such as clomipramine and the selective serotonin reuptake inhibitor (SSRI) fluoxetine, based on the assumption that trichotillomania is related to OCD and that such agents show selective efficacy in the treatment of OCD (Fineberg and Gale 2005).

The effects of the tricyclic agent clomipramine (50–250 mg/day) on hair pulling were compared with those of the tricyclic desipramine (50–250 mg/day) in a 10-week double-blind, crossover design, following 2 weeks of single-blind placebo lead-in (Swedo et al. 1989). Clomipramine has predominant effects on serotonin, whereas desipramine is relatively noradrenergic in its mechanisms. There were 13 recruits (all women), all of whom completed the study. Clomipramine showed clear superiority over desipramine, albeit there was no parallel placebo control arm to test whether desipramine showed any signs of efficacy.

Fluoxetine was subsequently tested in two small, randomized trials. Fluoxetine (20–80 mg/day) was compared with placebo in 15 subjects (14 [93.3%] women) in a 6-week double-blind, crossover study with a 5-week washout period between treatment arms (Christenson et al. 1991a). Fourteen (93.3%) of the 15 enrolled subjects completed the study. No significant differences were found between fluoxetine and placebo on primary outcome measures relating to hair-pulling symptoms.

In another study using a double-blind, placebo-controlled, crossover design, fluoxetine (20–80 mg) was evaluated over 31 weeks for 23 participants

(86.9% female). Sixteen of the 23 subjects (70%) completed the trial. The researchers found that fluoxetine failed to differentiate from placebo on primary outcome measures (Streichenwein and Thornby 1995).

Nonserotonergic drugs have also been evaluated for trichotillomania in randomized, blinded trials. O'Sullivan and Christenson (1999) performed a placebo-controlled, 6-week, randomized, double-blind, parallel study of the opioid antagonist naltrexone. Ten subjects received placebo and seven received naltrexone 50 mg/day. Nearly half of those taking naltrexone (compared with none on placebo) reduced hair pulling by more than 50%; however, two other measures of symptom improvement showed a nonsignificant change in the anticipated direction.

Grant et al. (2009) evaluated the glutamatergic agent N-acetylcysteine (1,200–2,400 mg/day) in the treatment of trichotillomania. This was a 12-week treatment trial using a double-blind, placebo-controlled design (50 subjects, 45 [90%] women). Fifty-six percent of patients were much or very much improved with active treatment, compared with 16% on placebo—a highly significant benefit of active treatment.

Most recently, the effects of the atypical antipsychotic olanzapine (2.5–20 mg/day) on trichotillomania symptoms were evaluated in a double-blind, placebo-controlled, parallel design for 12 weeks (25 participants, 17 [68%] of whom were female) (Van Ameringen et al. 2010). Eighty-five percent of those assigned to receive olanzapine, compared with 17% of those receiving placebo, improved during the trial, and this difference was highly significant statistically.

One trial has compared psychotherapy with pharmacological treatment in conjunction with a placebo arm in hair pullers (Ninan et al. 2000). The total sample size was 23 subjects, of which 16 (13 [81.3%] females) completed the trial. Subjects with trichotillomania were randomly assigned to nine weekly sessions of cognitive-behavioral therapy (CBT—a combination of habit reversal, stimulus control, and stress management; 7 subjects), clomipramine (up to 250 mg/day; 10 subjects), or placebo pill (6 subjects). CBT significantly reduced the severity of trichotillomania symptoms compared with clomipramine and placebo over the course of the study, whereas clomipramine and placebo did not differentiate from each other—arguably not surprising given the small sample size. There was no appropriate control for the CBT condition to evaluate specificity of content in moderating outcome.

Open-Label Trials

Two open-label studies were identified for trichotillomania, both involving SSRIs. In the first of such trials, fluoxetine (20–80 mg/day) was administered open-label for 7–12 weeks. Of the 17 recruits (16 of whom were women), 13 completed the trial (Koran et al. 1992). Severity of hair pulling decreased significantly over time for 9 of the 13 subjects (69.2%) as measured by reductions on the compulsions subscale of the Yale-Brown Obsessive Compulsive Scale.

van Minnen et al. (2003) investigated the efficacy of six sessions (12 weeks) of behavior therapy compared with fluoxetine (up to 60 mg/day) or a wait-list control group condition. Forty of the 43 participants completed the study (14 in behavior therapy, 11 in the fluoxetine group, and 15 in the wait-list group). The therapy group improved significantly more than the other groups during treatment, whereas drug treatment did not significantly differentiate from the wait-list control condition. A 2-year follow-up of the same patients suggested that the benefits of symptom improvement following therapy waned over time (Keijsers et al. 2006).

Case Reports

Published case reports have documented potential benefits from the following agents in trichotillomania: isocarboxazid (monoamine oxidase inhibitor [MAOI]), antipsychotics (haloperidol, olanzapine, risperidone, haloperidol, aripiprazole, quetiapine), serotonin reuptake inhibitors/SSRIs (clomipramine, sertraline, paroxetine, fluoxetine, fluvoxamine, escitalopram), inositol, lithium, bupropion, topiramate, riluzole, oxcarbazepine, trazodone, and naltrexone.

PATHOLOGICAL SKIN PICKING

Double-Blind Trials

There have been four pharmacological treatment trials in PSP with a double-blind component: three using SSRIs, and one using the mood stabilizer lamotrigine.

Fluoxetine (20–80 mg/day) was evaluated in 21 adults (16 [76.2%] women) with PSP in a 10-week double-blind, placebo-controlled study (Simeon et al. 1997). There were 4 noncompleters, yielding group sizes of 6 fluoxetine subjects and 11 placebo subjects. In both the completer and intent-to-treat analyses, fluoxetine showed superiority to placebo on a visual analogue scale outcome measure. On clinical global improvement, the completer analysis yielded a significant benefit of active versus placebo treatment, whereas this comparison did not obtain significance in the intent-to-treat analysis.

Bloch et al. (2001) undertook a complementary fluoxetine SSRI study (20–60 mg/day) in women with PSP who first received 6 weeks of open-label active treatment. The initial treatment responders (8 of 15 recruits) were then randomly assigned, in a double-blind manner, to fluoxetine or placebo for a further 6 weeks. Responders assigned to receive placebo (4 subjects) showed symptom worsening over time, whereas responders assigned to active treatment (4 subjects) showed sustained response; the comparison of percentage change from baseline to end point between placebo and active treatment was significant.

In addition, 45 subjects with PSP (32 [71.1%] women) were randomly assigned to receive an alternative SSRI, fixed-dose citalopram (20 mg/day; 23 subjects), or placebo (22 subjects) in a 4-week double-blind, parallel design (Arbabi et al. 2008). There were 20 citalopram and 20 placebo completers. Both citalopram and placebo were associated with significant improvements on symptom and quality-of-life measures, and the citalopram group showed significantly greater improvements than the placebo group (these appeared to be according to intent-to-treat analyses, although this was not made explicit). No significant differences, however, were observed between groups in terms of visual analogue scale scores.

Grant et al. (2010) undertook a double-blind, placebo-controlled trial with lamotrigine in 35 people with PSP (29 [82.9%] women). There were 25 completers, with 12 randomly assigned to receive lamotrigine and 13 to receive placebo. Active and placebo treatment did not significantly differentiate from each other on primary outcome measures. Interestingly, patients assigned to active treatment who showed relatively impaired baseline cognitive function (set-shifting and response inhibition) exhibited the most treatment response. The authors suggested that the lamotrigine response in PSP may unmask relevant neurobiological heterogeneity underpinning the disorder.

Open-Label Trials

There have been three open-label treatment trials in PSP: two with SSRIs and one with lamotrigine.

Treatment with the SSRI fluvoxamine (50–300 mg/day) was explored in a 12-week open-label study involving 14 female outpatients with neurotic skin excoriation (Arnold et al. 1999), 7 of whom completed the trial. Treatment was associated with significant improvements in skin excoriation but not depressive measures. In an 18-week open-label trial of escitalopram (10–30 mg/day) in 29 subjects (24 women) with PSP, treatment was associated with significant improvements on primary symptom outcome measures (Keuthen et al. 2007). There were 19 completers, and subjects had undertaken a 2-week placebo run-in prior to receiving the escitalopram.

Grant et al. (2007b) explored the effects of lamotrigine (25–300 mg/day) on symptoms of PSP in 24 subjects (19 [79.2%] women). This was a 12-week open-label study with 20 completers (last-observation-carried-forward approach). It was found that PSP symptoms, including urges to pick and actual picking behavior, improved significantly over time in the majority of subjects.

Case Reports

Published case reports have documented potential benefits from the following agents in PSP: serotonin reuptake inhibitors/SSRIs (fluoxetine, paroxetine), inositol, naltrexone, riluzole, olanzapine, topiramate, and paliperidone (serotonin receptor [5-HT]/dopamine$_2$ [D$_2$] antagonist).

PATHOLOGICAL NAIL BITING (ONYCHOPHAGIA)

Double-Blind Trials

There has been only one controlled pharmacological trial for the treatment of onychophagia. Leonard et al. (1991) examined the effects of clomipramine (mean dosage, 120 mg/day; range, 25–250 mg/day) and desipramine (135 mg/day; range, 25–250 mg/day) on nail biting in 25 adult subjects (age range, 21–42 years; 19 women). This study had a 2-week placebo run-in (1 subject was excluded as a placebo responder), followed by a 5-week crossover with each agent. There were 14 completers. Significantly greater clinical improvement was seen with clomipramine than with desipramine in nail biting but not in depression or on anxiety measures. There was no parallel placebo control arm.

Open-Label Trials

No open-label pharmacological trials for pathological nail biting have been reported.

Case Studies

Published case reports have documented potential benefits from the following agents in onychophagia: *N*-acetylcysteine, topiramate, bupropion, and fluoxetine.

SUMMARY OF PHARMACOLOGICAL EVIDENCE FOR THE TREATMENT OF GROOMING DISORDERS

Although there are many promising case reports on potential pharmacological treatments for trichotillomania, PSP, and onychophagia, positive data from controlled trials are sparse indeed.

For trichotillomania, there was limited positive evidence from controlled studies to support the utility of naltrexone, *N*-acetylcysteine, and olanzapine in its treatment (all category B evidence, recommendation grade 3, according to the guideline by Bandelow et al. [2008]; see Table 12–1, based on evidence hierarchy of Eccles and Mason [2001]; see Figure 12–1). (See Table 12–2 for a summary of recommendations by disorder.) Findings with clomipramine were inconsistent (category D evidence, recommendation grade 5), although it is likely that the single negative placebo-controlled trial ($n=23$) was underpowered, whereas adequate studies proving efficacy or nonefficacy of fluoxetine are lacking (category F evidence). There was some evidence from one or more case reports to support the potential utility of the following agents in treating trichotillomania (class C2 evidence, recommendation grade 4): isocarboxazid (MAOI), antipsychotics (haloperidol, olanzapine, risperidone, aripiprazole, quetiapine), serotonin reuptake inhibitors/SSRIs (sertraline, paroxetine, fluvoxamine, escitalopram), inositol, lithium, bupropion, topiramate, riluzole, oxcarbazepine, and trazodone.

For PSP, fluoxetine may be considered as a treatment with full evidence of efficacy (category A evidence, recommendation grade 1), although one of the positive placebo-referenced trials tested relapse prevention in a more limited subsample of fluoxetine responders. There was also limited positive evidence to support citalopram (category B evidence, recommendation grade 3), whereas fluvoxamine and escitalopram showed lesser evidence (category C1 evidence, recommendation grade 4). There was one negative double-blind study of lamotrigine that may have been underpowered ($n=35$), but an openlabel study was positive, suggesting ambiguity (category F evidence, i.e., lack of adequate evidence overall). There was also evidence from one or more case reports to support the potential utility of the following agents in treating PSP (class C2 evidence, recommendation grade 4): paroxetine, inositol, naltrexone, riluzole, olanzapine, topiramate, and paliperidone (5-HT/D$_2$ antagonist).

For onychophagia, clomipramine showed limited positive evidence from a controlled study based on a crossover trial showing superiority versus desipramine (category B evidence, recommendation grade 3). There was also evidence from one or more case reports to support the potential utility of the following agents in treating pathological nail biting (class C2 evidence, recommendation grade 4): N-acetylcysteine, topiramate, bupropion, and fluoxetine.

METHODOLOGICAL SHORTCOMINGS

Several methodological issues should be considered in supporting the pharmacological treatment evidence for grooming disorders. Studies were limited by the small sample sizes, thus constraining power to detect treatment effects versus stringent control conditions. In general terms, for a within-subject crossover design, the numbers of participants needed to achieve greater than 80% power to detect a significant drug effect with effect sizes of 0.2, 0.5, and 0.7, respectively, are 199, 34, and 19 participants (two-tailed test, *P*-value threshold of 0.05). As such, most trials were underpowered to detect small and medium effects of active treatment compared with placebo, meaning that null findings should be regarded with caution prior to larger trials being conducted to yield firm "negative" evidence. In those studies showing clinical benefits of treatments, long-term follow-up data were sparse. The positive crossover trials for clomipramine (trichotillomania and onychophagia) did not have a parallel placebo treatment arm to contextualize the findings. Finally, heterogeneity exists between trials in the diagnosis/definition of trichotillomania, PSP, and onychophagia; the occurrence of comorbidities; the treatment duration; and the instruments used for primary outcome measures. As such, the findings from individual trials may not generalize. In relation to treatment duration, longer-term studies are needed to see if treatment effects endure.

NEUROBIOLOGICAL MODELS

Neurobiological approaches have provided new insights into brain circuitry, neurotransmitters, and cognitive functions implicated in the pathophysiology of the aberrant grooming disorders considered herein. Of the published studies, most studies have been conducted in trichotillomania patients. Trichotillomania, PSP, and onychophagia can be considered pathological grooming behaviors involving dysfunction of cortico-subcortical neural circuitry involved in affect regulation, behavioral addiction, and cognitive control (Grant et al. 2007a). Cognitive and neuroimaging findings in people with trichotillomania have been reviewed in depth elsewhere (Chamberlain et al. 2007, 2009b; see also Chapter 4). Regions implicated in trichotillomania, based on structural imaging findings in comparisons with healthy control subjects, include the right frontal cortex, anterior cingulate cortices, and putamen (Chamberlain et al. 2010). Together these regions constitute a putative circuit that is responsible for generating motor habits and suppressing them (Aron et al. 2007; Hampshire et al. 2010). Other implicated regions include the amygdalo-hippocampal formation (involved in mood regulation and aspects of memory) and cerebellum (involved in motor learning). It is probable that similar regions are involved in PSP and onychophagia, although there have been no imaging studies as yet.

Consistent with dysregulation of neural circuitry involved in response suppression in grooming disorders, several studies have identified impaired response inhibition in patients. On the stop-signal task, subjects observe a series of directional arrows appearing on a computer screen one at a time and

TABLE 12–1.   Categories of evidence and summary of recommendations

Category	Description	Based on
A (↑↑)	Full evidence from controlled studies	Two or more double-blind, parallel-group RCTs showing superiority to placebo (or in the case of psychotherapy studies, superiority to a "psychological placebo" in a study with adequate blinding), *and*
		One or more positive RCTs showing superiority to or equivalent efficacy compared with established comparator treatment in a three-arm study with placebo control or in a well-powered non-inferiority trial (only required if such a standard treatment exists)
		In the case of existing negative studies (studies showing nonsuperiority to placebo or inferiority to comparator treatment), these must be outweighed by at least two more positive studies or a meta-analysis of all available studies that shows superiority to placebo and non-inferiority to an established comparator treatment.
B (↑)	Limited positive evidence from controlled studies	One or more RCTs showing superiority to placebo (or in the case of psychotherapy studies, superiority to a "psychological placebo"), *or*
		A randomized, controlled comparison with a standard treatment without placebo control with a sample size sufficient for a non-inferiority trial, *and*
		No negative studies exist
C (↑)	Evidence from uncontrolled studies or case reports/ expert opinion	
C1	Uncontrolled studies	One or more positive naturalistic open studies (with a minimum of five evaluable patients), *or*
		A comparison with a reference drug with a sample size insufficient for a non-inferiority trial, *and*
		No negative controlled studies exist

TABLE 12–1. Categories of evidence and summary of recommendations (*continued*)

Category	Description	Based on
C (↑) (*continued*)	Evidence from uncontrolled studies or case reports/expert opinion	
C2	Case reports	One or more positive case reports, *and* No negative controlled studies exist
C3		The opinion of experts in the field or clinical experience
D (↔)	Inconsistent results	Positive RCTs are outweighed by an approximately equal number of negative studies
E (↓)	Negative evidence	Majority of RCTs show nonsuperiority to placebo (or in the case of psychotherapy studies, superiority to a "psychological placebo") or inferiority to comparator treatment
F (?)	Lack of evidence	Adequate studies proving efficacy or nonefficacy are lacking

Recommendation grade	Based on
1	Category A evidence *and* good risk–benefit ratio
2	Category A evidence *and* moderate risk–benefit ratio
3	Category B evidence
4	Category C evidence
5	Category D evidence

Source.   Reprinted from Bandelow B, Zohar J, Hollander E, et al.: "World Federation of Societies of Biological Psychiatry (WFSBP) Guidelines for the Pharmacological Treatment of Anxiety, Obsessive-Compulsive and Post-traumatic Stress Disorders—First Revision." *World Journal of Biological Psychiatry* 9:248–312, 2008. Copyright 2008, World Federation of Societies of Biological Psychiatry.

TABLE 12–2. Summary of recommendations

Category/ Recommendation grade	Medication (listed alphabetically)
Trichotillomania	
B/3	*N*-Acetylcysteine, naltrexone, olanzapine
C2/4	Aripiprazole, bupropion, escitalopram, fluvoxamine, haloperidol, inositol, isocarboxazid, lithium, olanzapine, oxcarbazepine, paroxetine, quetiapine, riluzole, risperidone, sertraline, topiramate, trazodone
D/5	Clomipramine
F	Fluoxetine
Pathological skin picking	
A/1	Fluoxetine
B/3	Citalopram
C1/4	Escitalopram, fluvoxamine
C2/4	Inositol, naltrexone, olanzapine, paliperidone, paroxetine, riluzole, topiramate
F	Lamotrigine
Onychophagia	
B/3	Clomipramine
C2/4	Bupropion, fluoxetine, *N*-acetylcysteine, topiramate

Source. Adapted from Bandelow B, Zohar J, Hollander E, et al.: "World Federation of Societies of Biological Psychiatry (WFSBP) Guidelines for the Pharmacological Treatment of Anxiety, Obsessive-Compulsive and Post-traumatic Stress Disorders—First Revision." *World Journal of Biological Psychiatry* 9:248–312, 2008. Copyright 2008, World Federation of Societies of Biological Psychiatry.

attempt to stop their responses whenever a stop-signal (e.g., auditory beep) occurs. By varying the timing between the presentation of the directional arrow and occurrence of the stop-signal dynamically, this task provides an estimate of the time taken by the volunteer's brain to suppress responses, referred to as the *stop-signal reaction time.* Compared with control subjects, we have identified impaired reaction times in trichotillomania and PSP patients (Chamberlain et al. 2006; Odlaug et al. 2010). The precise neural "locus" of

Level	Type of evidence	
		Highest-level evidence, typically fewer studies
I	Evidence from a single randomized controlled trial or a meta-analysis of randomized controlled trials	
IIa	Evidence from at least one well-designed controlled study without randomization or with potential bias (e.g., randomized design using "initial treatment" responders only)	
IIb	Evidence from at least one other well-designed quasi-experimental study (e.g., open-label studies)	
III	Evidence from well-designed nonexperimental descriptive studies, such as comparative studies, correlation studies, and case studies	
IV	Evidence from expert committee reports or opinions and/or clinical experiences of respected authorities	
		Lowest-level evidence, typically more studies

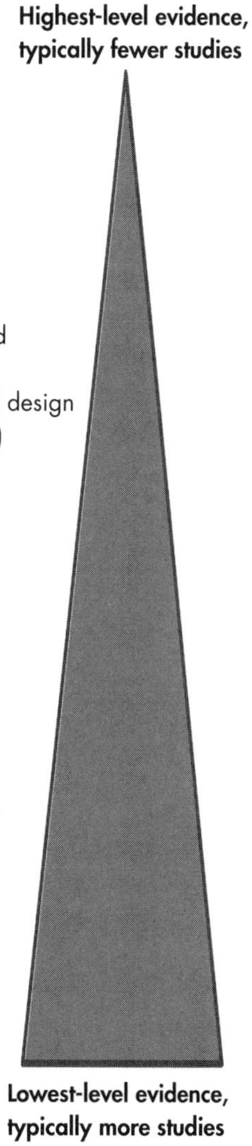

FIGURE 12–1. Evidence hierarchy.

Although not considered in the figure, pharmacological evidence from preclinical studies may also be considered, because this may suggest novel treatment directions and help to elucidate treatment mechanisms.

Source. Adapted from Eccles and Mason 2001.

these behavioral impairments is not yet known: it may be that the deficit is driven by overzealous basal ganglia activity (likely dopaminergic influence) or a lack of right frontal activity (likely noradrenergic influence).

In view of the available neurobiological data, we speculate that pharmacological treatments may wish to target the dissociable aspects of these body-focused repetitive behaviors, or grooming disorders. The addictive aspect of grooming behaviors may respond to agents such as N-acetylcysteine and naltrexone, whereas anxious/depressive features may respond to serotonin reuptake inhibitors (e.g., clomipramine); impulsive symptoms and sleep disruption due to these disorders (where present) may respond best to agents such as atomoxetine—medications capable of augmenting inhibitory control dependent on right frontal activity (Chamberlain et al. 2009a). Future work is needed to evaluate these predictions.

GUIDING CLINICIANS: THE TAKE-HOME MESSAGE

Our systematic review of the evidence supporting pharmacotherapies for trichotillomania, PSP, and onychophagia reveals a lamentable shortage of adequate studies upon which to base firm treatment recommendations. Nonetheless, there is probably sufficient evidence from randomized, controlled trials to support the use of naltrexone, N-acetylcysteine, and olanzapine for patients with trichotillomania, the SSRIs fluoxetine and citalopram for PSP, and clomipramine for nail biting.

In light of the likely neurobiological overlap across these disorders, clinicians and patients may consider that the relatively low adverse-effect profile associated with SSRIs, such as fluoxetine or citalopram, and perhaps even the serotonin reuptake inhibitor clomipramine, may still warrant a trial of their use as first-line agents for all three disorders as well as further evaluation in trials. Agents respectively associated, in some patients, with metabolic effects and liver dysfunction—namely, olanzapine and naltrexone—may therefore be regarded currently as second-line treatments. Moreover, current prescribing difficulties for N-acetylcysteine, related to the fact that it is not a regulated pharmacological product, limit its practical provision by clinicians in many countries at the present time. Properly powered double-blind trials with long-term follow-up are sorely needed to examine these and other potentially beneficial pharmacological treatments before firm treatment algorithms can be generated.

REFERENCES

American Psychiatric Association: Diagnosis and Statistical Manual of Mental Disorders, 4th Edition, Text Revision. Washington, DC, American Psychiatric Association, 2000

Arbabi M, Farnia V, Balighi K, et al: Efficacy of citalopram in the treatment of pathological skin picking: a randomized double blind placebo controlled trial. Acta Med Iran 46:367–372, 2008

Arnold LM, McElroy SL, Mutasim DF, et al: Characteristics of 34 adults with psychogenic excoriation. J Clin Psychiatry 59:509–514, 1998

Arnold LM, Mutasim DF, Dwight MM, et al: An open clinical trial of fluvoxamine treatment of psychogenic excoriation. J Clin Psychopharmacol 19:15–18, 1999

Aron AR, Behrens TE, Smith S, et al: Triangulating a cognitive control network using diffusion-weighted MRI and functional MRI. J Neurosci 27:3743–3752, 2007

Bandelow B, Zohar J, Hollander E, et al: World Federation of Societies of Biological Psychiatry (WFSBP) guidelines for the pharmacological treatment of anxiety, obsessive-compulsive and post-traumatic stress disorders—first revision. World J Biol Psychiatry 9:248–312, 2008

Bloch MR, Elliott M, Thompson H, et al: Fluoxetine in pathologic skin-picking: open-label and double-blind results. Psychosomatics 42:314–319, 2001

Bohne A, Keuthen N, Wilhelm S: Pathologic hairpulling, skin picking, and nail biting. Ann Clin Psychiatry 17:227–232, 2005

Chamberlain SR, Fineberg NA, Blackwell AD, et al: Motor inhibition and cognitive flexibility in obsessive-compulsive disorder and trichotillomania. Am J Psychiatry 163:1282–1284, 2006

Chamberlain SR, Menzies LA, Sahakian BJ, et al: Lifting the veil on trichotillomania. Am J Psychiatry 164:568–574, 2007

Chamberlain SR, Hampshire A, Müller U, et al: Atomoxetine modulates right inferior frontal activation during inhibitory control: a pharmacological functional magnetic resonance imaging study. Biol Psychiatry 65:550–555, 2009a

Chamberlain SR, Odlaug BL, Boulougouris V, et al: Trichotillomania: neurobiology and treatment. Neurosci Biobehav Rev 33:831–842, 2009b

Chamberlain SR, Hampshire A, Menzies L, et al: Reduced white matter integrity in trichotillomania: a diffusion tensor imaging study. Arch Gen Psychiatry 67:965–971, 2010

Christenson GA, Mackenzie TB, Mitchell JE, et al: A placebo-controlled, double-blind crossover study of fluoxetine in trichotillomania. Am J Psychiatry 148:1566–1571, 1991a

Christenson GA, Pyle RL, Mitchell JE: Estimated lifetime prevalence of trichotillomania in college students. J Clin Psychiatry 52:415–417, 1991b

Cullen BA, Samuels JF, Bienvenu OJ, et al: The relationship of pathologic skin picking to obsessive-compulsive disorder. J Nerv Ment Dis 189:193–195, 2001

Eccles M, Mason J: How to develop cost-conscious guidelines. Health Technol Assess 5:1–69, 2001

Fineberg NA, Gale TM: Evidence-based pharmacotherapy of obsessive-compulsive disorder. Int J Neuropsychopharmacol 8:107–129, 2005

Franklin ME, Flessner CA, Woods DW, et al: The Child and Adolescent Trichotillomania Impact Project: descriptive psychopathology, comorbidity, functional impairment, and treatment utilization. J Dev Behav Pediatr 29:493–500, 2008

Grant JE, Mancebo MC, Pinto A, et al: Impulse control disorders in adults with obsessive compulsive disorder. J Psychiatr Res 40:494–501, 2006

Grant JE, Odlaug BL, Kim SW: Lamotrigine treatment of pathologic skin picking: an open-label study. J Clin Psychiatry 68:1384–1391, 2007a

Grant JE, Odlaug BL, Potenza MN: Addicted to hair pulling? How an alternate model of trichotillomania may improve treatment outcome. Harv Rev Psychiatry 15:80–85, 2007b

Grant JE, Odlaug BL, Kim SW: N-Acetylcysteine, a glutamate modulator, in the treatment of trichotillomania: a double-blind, placebo-controlled study. Arch Gen Psychiatry 66:756–763, 2009

Grant JE, Odlaug BL, Chamberlain SR, et al: A double-blind, placebo-controlled trial of lamotrigine for pathologic skin picking: treatment efficacy and neurocognitive predictors of response. J Clin Psychopharmacol 30:396–403, 2010

Hampshire A, Chamberlain SR, Monti MM, et al: The role of the right inferior frontal gyrus: inhibition and attentional control. Neuroimage 50:1313–1319, 2010

Hayes SL, Storch EA, Berlanga L: Skin picking behaviors: an examination of the prevalence and severity in a community sample. J Anxiety Disord 23:314–319, 2009

Hollander E, Kim S, Khanna S, et al: Obsessive-compulsive disorder and obsessive-compulsive spectrum disorders: diagnostic and dimensional issues. CNS Spectr 12(suppl):5–13, 2007

Keijsers GP, van Minnen A, Hoogduin CA, et al: Behavioural treatment of trichotillomania: two-year follow-up results. Behav Res Ther 44:359–370, 2006

Keuthen NJ, Jameson M, Loh R, et al: Open-label escitalopram treatment for pathological skin picking. Int Clin Psychopharmacol 22:268–274, 2007

Keuthen NJ, Koran LM, Aboujaoude E, et al: The prevalence of pathologic skin picking in US adults. Compr Psychiatry 51:183–186, 2010

King RA, Zohar AH, Ratzoni G, et al: An epidemiological study of trichotillomania in Israeli adolescents. J Am Acad Child Adolesc Psychiatry 34:1212–1215, 1995

Koran LM, Ringold A, Hewlett W: Fluoxetine for trichotillomania: an open clinical trial. Psychopharmacol Bull 28:145–149, 1992

Leonard HL, Lenane MC, Swedo SE, et al: A double-blind comparison of clomipramine and desipramine treatment of severe onychophagia (nail biting). Arch Gen Psychiatry 48:821–827, 1991

Ninan PT, Rothbaum BO, Marsteller FA, et al: A placebo-controlled trial of cognitive-behavioral therapy and clomipramine in trichotillomania. J Clin Psychiatry 61:47–50, 2000

Odlaug BL, Grant JE: Childhood-onset pathologic skin picking: clinical characteristics and psychiatric comorbidity. Compr Psychiatry 48:388–393, 2007

Odlaug BL, Grant JE: Trichotillomania and pathologic skin picking: clinical comparison with an examination of comorbidity. Ann Clin Psychiatry 20:57–63, 2008

Odlaug BL, Grant JE: Impulse-control disorders in a college sample. Prim Care Companion J Clin Psychiatry 12(2), 2010

Odlaug BL, Chamberlain SR, Grant JE: Motor inhibition and cognitive flexibility in pathologic skin picking. Prog Neuropsychopharmacol Biol Psychiatry 34:208–211, 2010

O'Sullivan RL, Christenson GA: Pharmacotherapy of trichotillomania, in Trichotillomania. Edited by Stein DJ, Christenson GA, Hollander E. Washington, DC, American Psychiatric Press, 1999, pp 93–124

Simeon D, Stein DJ, Gross S, et al: A double-blind trial of fluoxetine in pathologic skin picking. J Clin Psychiatry 58:341–347, 1997

Stein DJ, Chamberlain SR, Fineberg N: An A-B-C model of habit disorders: hair-pulling, skin-picking, and other stereotypic conditions. CNS Spectr 11:824–827, 2006

Stein DJ, Garner JP, Keuthen NJ, et al: Trichotillomania, stereotypic movement disorder, and related disorders. Curr Psychiatry Rep 9:301–302, 2007

Stein DJ, Flessner CA, Franklin M, et al: Is trichotillomania a stereotypic movement disorder? An analysis of body-focused repetitive behaviors in people with hair-pulling. Ann Clin Psychiatry 20:194–198, 2008

Streichenwein SM, Thornby JI: A long-term, double-blind, placebo-controlled crossover trial of the efficacy of fluoxetine for trichotillomania. Am J Psychiatry 152:1192–1196, 1995

Swedo SE, Leonard HL: Trichotillomania: an obsessive compulsive spectrum disorder? Psychiatr Clin North Am 15:777–790, 1992

Swedo SE, Leonard HL, Rapoport JL, et al: A double-blind comparison of clomipramine and desipramine in the treatment of trichotillomania (hair pulling). N Engl J Med 321:497–501, 1989

Van Ameringen M, Mancini C, Patterson B, et al: A randomized, double-blind, placebo-controlled trial of olanzapine in the treatment of trichotillomania. J Clin Psychiatry 71:1336–1343, 2010

van Minnen A, Hoogduin KA, Keijsers GP, et al: Treatment of trichotillomania with behavioral therapy or fluoxetine: a randomized, waiting-list controlled study. Arch Gen Psychiatry 60:517–522, 2003

Wilhelm S, Keuthen NJ, Deckersbach T, et al: Self-injurious skin picking: clinical characteristics and comorbidity. J Clin Psychiatry 60:454–459, 1999

Woods DW, Flessner CA, Franklin ME, et al: The Trichotillomania Impact Project (TIP): exploring phenomenology, functional impairment, and treatment utilization. J Clin Psychiatry 67:1877–1888, 2006

FAMILY INVOLVEMENT IN THE TREATMENT OF CHILDREN WITH BODY-FOCUSED REPETITIVE BEHAVIORS

Suzanne Mouton-Odum, Ph.D.
Ruth G. Golomb, M.Ed., LCPC

After one has read the previous 12 chapters of this book, it is probably clear that the body of research on hair pulling and skin picking is minimal at best and that additional information is greatly needed. Researchers are only at the beginning of understanding the etiology, phenomenology, and treatment of these body-focused repetitive behaviors (BFRBs), but they are trying resolutely to glean answers. There is virtually no empirical research on the efficacy of strategies that involve the family in treatment. As a result, this chapter is a bit different than the previous ones. The information provided here is based on clinical interactions with thousands of families, not on empirical research (Mouton-Odum and Golomb 2009). Nevertheless, the information provided is both important and necessary for the successful treatment of children and adolescents in the context of the systems in which they live.

In the treatment of children and adolescents with trichotillomania or skin picking, it is not only valuable but very often necessary to involve the family. In fact, in treatment with young people, family participation is often the most critical ingredient in the success or failure of the treatment process. In this chapter we describe positive ways to involve family members in treatment and illustrate how parents can be invaluable to the therapeutic process.

We begin by presenting a clear understanding of the unique experience of a parent whose child is pulling his or her hair or picking his or her skin. Second, we outline ways to educate parents about BFRBs by reviewing common questions, fears, and mistaken beliefs that can lead parents to engage in maladaptive responses. Third, we review some common mistakes that parents make when trying to help their child stop pulling his or her hair or picking his or her skin. Fourth, we provide specific ways for the reader to help parents correct these mistakes, thus teaching them to be helpful, not hurtful. Fifth, we present an overview of how the age and developmental level of the child dictate a parent's role and level of involvement in the therapy process. Finally, we cover slips and relapse, providing the reader with an understanding of how to help parents to appreciate treatment as a process that may involve forward and backward movement. In addition, we briefly address the role of a spouse when a member of the couple is engaged in a BFRB. It is our hope that the reader will use the information included in this chapter to help families begin to heal and approach their loved one's hair-pulling or skin-picking behavior in a more accepting and healthy way. In so doing, the therapist is in the unique position of helping families avoid a lifetime of shame, heartbreak, and anger, which commonly develop when these behaviors are not fully understood or adequately addressed.

UNDERSTANDING THE PARENTS' PERSPECTIVE

Typically, when a family presents for treatment of a BFRB, they are in crisis. Whether they have consulted with pediatricians or school counselors previously or the therapist is the first professional consultation, parents have almost always experienced frustration, anxiety, or even anger toward their child regarding these behaviors. It is important for treatment providers to have a good understanding of the parents' perspective so that they can validate the parents' feelings throughout the course of treatment.

When parents first notice their child's pulling or picking behavior—and, more importantly, the result of the pulling or picking (bald spots, scabs, or sores)—they initially experience fear. Parents generally do not understand this seemingly self-destructive behavior and usually respond with some form of "Stop it!" "Don't do that to yourself!" or "Quit!" In an attempt to eliminate this behavior, they will become quite attuned to their child's every movement, will scrutinize the child's appearance, and will remind the child to "put your hand down" when they see the behavior or anything that approximates the behavior. As the pulling or picking continues, which it invariably does, parents feel more and more out of control and helpless. This enormous frustration leads to more persistent reminders and eventually feelings of desperation. What might begin as attempts at being helpful eventually turn into nagging, shaming, or even punishing. As a result, it is possible for some or all family members to feel overly responsible, exhausted, emotionally drained, hurt, confused, and above all, hopeless.

Given parents' state of crisis, anxiety, and trepidation, it is helpful to initiate treatment by taking an educational approach. Parents need to be given relevant information about BFRBs and to have their questions about these behaviors clearly answered. In addition to taking a structured, psychoeducational approach, it is also helpful to normalize any feelings of fear and frustration. Just as individuals with BFRBs may feel isolated and ashamed, parents may also feel a unique loneliness and lack of support. In addition, parents may experience feelings of failure. In response, let parents know that their reactions and feelings are common and that most parents in their shoes react with virtually the same feelings and behaviors. Validating statements such as "You are probably very frightened and frustrated," "This feels really out of control," and "There is nothing worse than watching your child engage in this behavior and not being able to help them to stop" can be incredibly helpful to the parents and serve to reduce their anxiety about what is happening to their child.

It is important for the therapist, when working with families, to address common fears and questions that parents invariably have. Universal questions that almost all parents have in the beginning of treatment are as follows:

- What is this behavior?
- Why is this happening to my child?
- Did I cause this behavior—is it my fault?
- Will this go away?
- How many people have this?
- Why can't he or she stop?

A good portion of the first session should be spent educating parent(s) and child about the etiology, prevalence, and gender distribution of either trichotillomania or skin picking. It can be helpful to discuss this information with the child present and then again with the parents separately. This way, both child and parent(s) are receiving the same information at the same time but also have time alone with the therapist to address their own unique questions and feelings. Parents need to be reassured that these behaviors are similar to nail biting, are fairly common, and, although they tend to run in families, are not the result of a particular type of parenting and thus are not the parents' fault. Also, educating them about treatment can help decrease fears and reduce feelings of anxiety and hopelessness. It is helpful to conceptualize trichotillomania and skin picking as adaptive—that is, individuals engage in these behaviors because the behaviors are somehow helping to meet a need (emotional, sensory, physiological, or cognitive) (Mansueto et al. 1999). Throughout the process of therapy, a functional analysis is used to help understand how the BFRB is serving the child. After idiosyncratic needs are identified, alternative coping strategies are then explored. Parents come to understand that the BFRB is in some way meeting a unique need of the child (e.g., self-soothing, sensory stimulation, emotional regulation), and this helps to change the perception from one of blame to one of understanding.

The last question, "Why can't he or she stop?" is perhaps the most common and most confusing to parents. Some assumptions that may be underlying this question are that the child's behavior is purposeful, that the child is pulling or picking to punish the parent, and that the behavior is an attempt to make the child "ugly." Additionally, parents may assume that if their child really tried or really wanted to, he or she *could* stop. Addressing these assumptions early on can help parents understand that BFRBs are not completely voluntary, are not malicious or manipulative, and are not easily changed. Furthermore, explaining that these behaviors are based upon biological or possibly neurological functions can help parents develop a level of empathy and compassion for their child that did not previously exist. To address the question "Why can't he or she stop?" it is often helpful to use common examples of behaviors that are difficult to change. This is an excerpt from a therapy session in which the therapist is explaining why a patient cannot stop her behavior:

> All of us have tried to change behaviors in our lives. One that we can all relate to is eating junk food or sweets. We know that eating unhealthy foods will cause us to gain weight or will elevate our cholesterol, but we don't always make the right choices. Just knowing that eating the salad is better for me than the hamburger does not guarantee that I will order it. In fact, if my spouse tells me not to eat the hamburger because it will make me fat, I am even *more* inclined to order it. In other words, your child is pulling because in that moment it is making her feel better, even if she knows that she might regret it later. Telling her that she will regret it or that she should do something else might actually cause her to want to pull more.

So what are parents supposed to do to help their child? We make some specific suggestions later in this chapter about how parents can be helpful, but first it is important to review common mistaken beliefs about hair pulling and skin picking as well as common errors that parents make when approaching their child with a BFRB.

ADDRESSING MISTAKEN BELIEFS

It is not unusual for parents to present for treatment after having gotten mistaken information about BFRBs from the Internet or having been given such information from misinformed professionals or society in general. At the outset of treatment, the therapist should address common mistaken beliefs that contribute to parent confusion and fear so that fears based on these beliefs can be diminished. For example, parents are sometimes told that hair pulling or skin picking is the result of trauma that their child may have experienced. When parents hear this information, they may assume that the child has been a victim of some unknown abuse, leading to frightening thoughts, out-of-control feelings, and intense anxiety. Reassure parents that most children do not report any stressful situations occurring at the onset of a BFRB. There is no evidence in the literature to support the assumption of an abusive event leading to the onset of a BFRB.

Additionally, parents may feel blamed or blame themselves. They may fear that they are being perceived as "unfit" because of their child's "self-destructive" behavior. Parents may think or be told that their child must have some underlying inner conflict or "issue" that, if resolved, would cure the BFRB. This assertion is not supported in any of the literature regarding BFRBs. Educating parents about BFRBs and reiterating that the behaviors are not the result of trauma, poor parenting, or some underlying, unresolved conflict can help them to feel less defensive and angry about their child's behavior, thus promoting compassion and understanding.

Another mistaken belief is that hair pulling or skin picking will lead to some other, more pathological behavior such as self-mutilation or suicidal tendencies. The reality is that although BFRBs can be persistent, they do not lead to or predict any other future behaviors. A recent investigation by Franklin et al. (2008) showed that the incidence of comorbid psychological disorders among children with trichotillomania was no higher than that in the general population. Probably the most disturbing mistaken belief that parents often present with is that BFRBs are a form of self-mutilation and/or the result of a desire to harm the body. This belief not only is damaging to the patient but also can unnecessarily elevate fear among parents. It is important for clinicians to be very clear that BFRBs are not self-mutilation, but rather more like self-soothing or self-stimulating behaviors. For parents who do not pull hair or pick skin themselves, this may be difficult to comprehend. Using examples that parents may be more likely to relate to, such as eating unhealthy foods or smoking cigarettes, sometimes helps them to see how humans sometimes engage in behaviors that, although harmful long term, can be pleasurable in the present. Insight or knowing that a behavior is unhealthy does not guarantee that the behavior will diminish. How long have people known that smoking cigarettes is dangerous to one's health? Yet cigarette smoking still remains the most preventable cause of illness and death in the United States, despite this very clear information.

IDENTIFYING COMMON MISTAKES PARENTS MAKE

Common mistakes that parents typically make that should be addressed in therapy are impatience, blaming, policing, and too much focus.

Impatience leading to frustration is common for parents who are dealing with their child's BFRB. Therefore, in the beginning of treatment it is important to evaluate the readiness of the child or adolescent to be involved in the therapeutic process. All too often, it is the parents who are motivated for treatment, whereas the child is at best reluctant. Becoming impatient and trying to force children to participate in treatment, to give up their BFRBs before they are ready, can actually cause the behaviors to get worse. When parents are pushing treatment and the child is clearly not ready, it is recommended that therapy involve the parents only. There are a multitude of things that parents can work on to help their child feel less pressure without addressing the BFRB directly. These parent strategies will be outlined in the next section of this chapter. When a child or adolescent eventually does express interest in making change, parents are then in a much better position to assist in this process.

In the beginning, however, when parents are more motivated for treatment than their child, the parents will likely become frustrated. They will point out that they have sought out all of the strategies and made them readily available to their child and he or she "just won't use them!" Parents can become more than frustrated—they can become angry. It is important to help parents understand their child's ambivalence, if present, and to predict that the child will become aggravated if change is expected before he or she is ready. Discussing change as a process rather than an event can be useful when addressing the frustration many parents experience when they are eager to see change and the child is not quite ready.

The second common mistake that parents make is to blame their child for the BFRB. Blaming is often the result of the underlying assumption that "she could stop if she really wanted to," which leads to the belief that BFRBs are voluntary behaviors that are easy to control. Initially, parents may encourage their child to change the behavior by saying things like "You look so pretty with your scabs healed up" or "Your eyelashes are so long and beautiful when they are grown out." These statements may seem supportive; however, when a child is struggling, has scabs, or is lacking eyelashes, these statements are actually heard as "You are not pretty" and "Your eyelashes are not long and not beautiful." Consistent feedback such as this can lead to withdrawal and self-degradation in a developing child or adolescent. Most often, young people with BFRBs feel blamed, frustrated, misunderstood, and pushed. Helping parents understand and then manage their own feelings is a vital part of therapy. Coaching and guiding parents to enable them to focus on the behavior, rather than the resulting hair loss or scab, is essential.

The third common mistake that parents make is policing their child's behavior. Policing occurs when parents take on the role of attempting to manage their child's behavior by daily questioning, inspecting, noticing, and commenting about hair, skin, or nails. In more extreme cases, parents have been known to shame, humiliate, or even punish a child for engaging in a BFRB. As a result of policing, the child can begin to believe that his or her worth as a human being is dependent upon the presence or absence of hair, skin, or nails. However, not reminding, not nagging, and not policing may feel to the parents as if they are being negligent. The therapist should explain that it is normal for parents to go through a period of frustration and panic in the beginning but that policing causes children to feel confused and down on themselves. An excerpt from a therapy session illustrates this approach:

> You love your child and want the best for her. The last thing you want is to see your child teased or humiliated on the playground for having a bald spot on her head. I know that you are trying to be a good parent by paying attention to this problem; however, we are going to talk about different ways to attend to this at home that will feel better to you and your child.

Later in this chapter we outline other specific ways for parents to be helpful without policing.

The final common mistake that parents and sometimes therapists make when dealing with a child who has a BFRB is "too much focus." Focusing exclusively on hair pulling or skin picking, either at home or in treatment, neglects important aspects of a developing child or adolescent. When a child comes home with a great report card and a bald spot, the therapist should help parents focus on the hard work and excellent report card rather than seeing only the bald spot. Parents need support to enable them to see their child as multidimensional and unique. Hair pulling or skin picking may be a part of who the child is, but it does not define him or her as a person. In addition we, as clinicians, must be careful to evaluate and understand the child or adolescent client in the context of his or her life. The bald spot that we see may not be what is most troubling to our client. Children with BFRBs experience the same stresses that other children experience at the same developmental stage—namely, difficult relationships within the family, peer pressure, academic challenges, learning disabilities, friendship disruptions, and so on. Often in treatment, the BFRB may not even be discussed during a session, depending on what events have taken place in the client's life. Again, too much focus on a BFRB can incorrectly send the message that a physical characteristic (hair, skin, or nails) is the most important aspect of who the child is, when it is not. It is the therapist's challenge to balance the discussion of the needs and experiences of the budding individual with the management of this challenging behavior.

WORKING WITH PARENTS ON HOW TO BE HELPFUL

During work with families struggling with BFRBs, it is important to provide parents with specific, measurable objectives. After common struggles that parents typically face have been identified and feelings have been validated, the treating therapist should outline strategies for parents to employ with the child. The overarching goal for parents, however, is to develop empathy for their child while viewing him or her as a whole and complete person.

First, parents must learn to be patient with the therapy process. They may have to accept that they are more motivated for treatment than their child. The therapist should help parents learn to be patient and to view maintenance of behavior change as a long-term goal that should be tended to daily, over the years, not a "cure" that is achieved. Often the more insistent a parent is on change, the slower a child will be to make that change. Being patient and allowing the child to move at his or her own pace is a more supportive and nurturing approach that ultimately allows the child to take responsibility for his or her own actions—a far healthier alternative. How do parents become more patient when they are so very concerned about their child? The first step is to make sure that parents are taking care of themselves. Encourage parents to

1. Gather support and information about trichotillomania and skin picking through books and videos or online at www.trich.org, or by attending a Trichotillomania Learning Center conference or retreat.
2. Identify maladaptive feelings, beliefs, and reactions. Instruct parents to keep a daily log of their emotions and their reactions to the child's BFRB for 1 week. Enable parents to identify and understand their feelings so that they can develop good coping skills to better manage their emotional reactions during this process.
3. Create time for themselves to engage in activities that are pleasurable, particularly exercise and social support.

4. Learn specific emotional regulation skills for calming down. Teach parents to walk away when they feel like yelling, take deep breaths when they notice themselves getting upset, or distract themselves when they want to nag about picking or pulling.
5. Focus on the child's use of coping strategies rather than the resulting bald patch or scab. When parents understand that their child will be trying to employ strategies that are designed to interfere with the pulling or picking, then the focus can shift to supporting the child's use of those strategies.
6. Remember that therapy is a process and that their child may need to try numerous, varied strategies until he or she discovers the right combination that will work. Parents may need regular and consistent reinforcement of these ideas.

Understandably, parents need a lot of therapeutic support throughout treatment. One parent described her role in helping her daughter cope with trichotillomania as "providing a soft place for her to fall," which illustrates the acceptance, support, and nonjudgmental approach that can lead to healing for the entire family.

Second, parents must learn to recognize when they are blaming their child for the BFRB. The most important tool when addressing blame in therapy is to teach parents *acceptance*. Accepting that hair pulling or skin picking is a part of how their child copes with boredom, fatigue, or stress is a critical part of the treatment process. It is human nature to want to blame an event or a person when things go wrong, but in this case, there really is no one to blame. Help parents to understand that the BFRB is a part of their child but not the definition of who the child is. Sometimes parents believe that if they accept the BFRB, they are somehow condoning the behavior. The therapist should provide an environment in which parents feel free to express their feelings and gain support. Acceptance leads to healing, not to increases in the BFRB.

Third, parents must learn to avoid policing their child's behavior. This policing feels worse than nagging to a child because the child often feels confused, frustrated, and not always in control of his or her behavior. Policing can drive a wedge between the parent and child, causing permanent damage to the relationship. The solution here is to release the need to control the child and allow the child to take more responsibility for his or her behavior. When parents are constantly "on top of" their child's behavior, the child has no incentive or ability to take responsibility him- or herself. Older children are engaged in the developmental task of establishing independence from their parents. It is appropriate for them to find their own ways to approach and solve problems. Therefore, policing latency-aged children and adolescents is particularly ineffective and potentially disruptive to the evolving relationship with the parents. Parents of these children often find that policing increases conflict in the home and contributes to a breakdown in communication and erosion of trust between the parents and the child. Therapists can help parents come up with alternative statements such as "I love you whether or not you have hair," "I am here to help if you would like me to; otherwise, I will leave this to you," or "I am more worried about how you are feeling, rather than how you are doing with pulling." These statements take the pressure off the child and help him or her feel less judged.

Finally, parents who are too focused on hair/skin/nails must learn to shift the focus away from the BFRB to all of the wonderful things about their child. A developing child can erroneously learn that the most important thing about him- or herself is whether or not he or she is engaging in the BFRB. Encourage parents to explore and emphasize their child's strengths and interests. For example, if a child loves art, focus on art; if he loves football, focus on football; if she is good at writing, focus on writing. A shift in focus to these aspects of the child can lead to improved self-esteem, the development of the child's identity in these areas, and improved self-confidence.

TREATING CHILDREN OF DIFFERING AGES AND DEVELOPMENTAL STAGES

The final important piece to working with families with BFRBs is to understand how developmental differences in children affect parents' roles in treatment. For the very young child, ages 0–5 years, treatment often involves only the parents. It is appropriate for parents of these very young children to be more involved in treatment than they would be for a 14-year-old, mainly because children this young cannot comprehend their behavior (it just feels good) and, more importantly, are not able to understand when or how to use coping strategies. Parents should be asked to observe their child's BFRB, notice trigger situations, identify any co-occurring feelings, and observe any comorbid behaviors (such as thumb sucking). Note that parents often automatically assume that their child who is pulling or picking must be experiencing "too much stress." In children this young, the word *stress* is not usually an accurate description of a child's emotional experience. Therefore, if the parent comes in with reports of a child's "stress," you will need to ask the parent to describe the trigger situation and circumstances that preceded the BFRB. A good therapist will take into account that young children who become fatigued often engage in BFRBs to soothe or calm themselves. This fatigue is not an example of stress as we know it but rather a natural experience that creates discomfort for children.

Once a parent has gathered these data, the therapist is able to help formulate a functional analysis of the child's behavior and ultimately identify ways to alter the child's environment to either impede the BFRB or, alternatively, to satisfy the intrinsic need that the child is satisfying through the BFRB. An example of this might be the following: if a parent observes the child pulling when he or she is overly tired, the parent can put thin gloves on the child's hands when the child is falling asleep (making it hard to pull) and can help the child balance playtime activities with rest or downtime, thus preventing these situations in which the child is overtired. Understanding the circumstances that trigger the pulling or picking behaviors allows the therapist to suggest a number of different strategies that could be used to help the youngster.

Many young families experience significant life transitions. It is very important for therapy to help these families with those transitions while concurrently working on the BFRB. Moving, introducing a new sibling, and changing jobs are all common occurrences during this stage of life. During these life transitions, it is important for the family to work on developing more adaptive coping skills. Because treatment at this age so intensely involves working with parents, the family must be sure that there will be plenty of support and emotional resources available at that time. If a parent or family member is experiencing severe depression, extreme marital conflict, or anxiety that is incapacitating, it is crucial to attend to these problems first before undertaking treatment for the BFRB.

Although children between the ages of 6 and 11 years are becoming increasingly aware of their behavior and the consequences of their behavior, they are typically less concerned with hair loss or skin damage than those who have reached middle school. Treatment for children this age often includes working with an incentive system. The long-term goal of achieving hair growth, long nails, or smooth skin is often too distant from the actual behavior change to function as a positive reinforcer. Parents are often asked to help provide ideas for rewards. It is important to note that rewards are issued to children for employing appropriate coping strategies to resist pulling or picking, rather than rewarding behavior cessation. In addition, bolstering a child's self-esteem is also crucial at this stage. Teach parents to couple a tangible reward with a social reward, such as saying, "Great job using your strategies today—here is a sticker for your calendar" or "I can see that you are trying really hard! Way to go!" In this way, the parent is reinforcing the child's effort, rewarding successful use of strategies, and providing positive, supportive comments that assist the child in the therapeutic process. As a result, the child begins to feel better about him- or herself and is less focused on bald spots or scabs. This shift often encourages children to talk about their progress and their struggles with the BFRB.

Children at this stage (ages 6–11 years) more than anything need to feel loved and accepted. Anxiety is common during the elementary school years; therefore, the goal of treatment is not to eliminate anxiety but to help the child develop better coping skills when anxious feelings inevitably arise. With regard to BFRBs at this age, parents are quite involved, but less so than those parents of preschool and toddler-aged children. Parents can be particularly helpful by modeling appropriate responses to disappointment, frustration, and even success regarding the BFRB. For example, when a child grows eyelashes, the parent is often invited by the child to comment on the new growth and the child's general appearance. Parents should be cautioned not to comment on "how good you look" as a result of reductions in the BFRB, but rather "how hard you must be working." Comments about appearance can backfire and are heard as "how bad you look when you don't have hair [or skin]." The therapist may predict slips in maintaining the behavior and instruct parents to respond to hair growth by commenting positively about the child's use of strategies: "I can see that you are working very hard on using your strategies. Great job! Let's talk about what is working." Focusing on the use of strategies rather than the successful hair growth or smooth skin can help parents gain a different perspective and alter emotional reactions. In addition, evaluating which strategies work and which do not helps prepare both parents and children for potential slips. When parents achieve perspective and control over their emotional reactivity, they are better able to model appropriate reactions to slips or disappointments.

Middle school is a time of tremendous change for children, both physically and emotionally. In treatment, the types of strategies selected and level of parent involvement will depend largely upon the child's temperament, maturity, and relationship with his or her parents. Some early adolescents are happy to have their parents involved in helping them, whereas other children at this age feel the need for greater independence from their parents. As a therapist, you can help negotiate how much parent involvement is going to be helpful to the child. Furthermore, middle school is typically the time when children begin to experience teasing from their peers as a result of hair pulling, skin picking, and other, non-BFRB, reasons. Although parents typically try to shelter their children from these negative experiences, let parents know that sometimes teasing can serve as a motivator for behavior change and can move a previously unwilling child into readiness.

Children at this developmental stage need to be in charge of dictating how involved their parents will be in treatment. If a child says "I do not want my mom to ask me about my hair," instruct the parent to keep quiet and to let you be in charge of hair questions. Again, this can be quite difficult for some parents and may require separate therapy sessions for one or both parents. Parents want to feel involved in treatment and to feel like they are actively helping their child. However, sometimes the best way for them to actively help is to not talk about hair pulling or skin picking at all. Parents need help and guidance about appropriate boundaries and respecting their child's wishes. In addition, children need to have the freedom to change their minds regarding their parents' involvement. One week a child may want his or her parent to stay completely out of the picture, and another week the same child may want the parent to provide cues or reminders to use certain strategies. The therapist will need to assist both parent and child to be flexible with making these ongoing changes.

High school years bring unique challenges that can be terribly complicated with the addition of a BFRB. Teenagers can be defiant and angry by nature. A great challenge that parents of adolescents face is how to manage their child's unpleasant behaviors without damaging the relationship. The most common mistake that parents of adolescents with BFRBs make is to allow hair pulling/skin picking to become a point of contention with their child—another battle in the war of adolescence. It is the therapist's job to help parents let their child take responsibility for the BFRB. In other words, parents must allow their child to pull or to pick without reaction or consequence. This can be very difficult for many parents. In other words, help parents let their child experience the consequences of the BFRB, while they remain neutral. What this looks like in many cases is ignoring obvious pulling/picking episodes. If a child comes home from school with a bald patch and the parent simply states, "How was your day?" it allows the child to share, if he or she wishes, how things went. In addition, there are no assumptions, judgments, criticisms, or negative statements involved.

Another common difficulty for parents of older adolescents is that they will avoid doling out punishment for misbehavior because they are afraid it will lead to increased pulling/picking. Avoiding deserved punishment is dangerous because it allows the adolescent to be in control and not suffer necessary consequences to poor behavior, possibly resulting in more maladaptive behavior. In addition, avoiding consequences may contribute to low self-esteem for the teen. Adolescents generally have an idea when their behavior is out of line. When parents resist enforcing appropriate behavior and do not give consequences, the teenager may begin to feel damaged, as if he or she is too "ill" to engage in reasonable behavior. Treating an adolescent delicately may lead to feelings of inadequacy and depression. The therapist should not allow the fear of hair pulling to prevent parents from giving appropriate and deserved consequences. In addition, the consequences of pulling or picking (bald spots, scabs, sores, and short nails) should be experienced by the adolescent, not the parent. If a mom is crying and feeling devastated by her daughter's bald spot, the child feels increased control, pressure, and responsibility for her mother's feelings, all of which are inappropriate for her development. It is the therapist's job to help parents take a backseat to their child's BFRB, allowing the child to step up to the plate for behavior change.

For treatment at any age, an incentive system is often quite useful. Even though adolescents and older teens are cognitively able to understand the short- and long-term consequences to their behavior, it is still quite a distance from the initial behavior change to the "reward" of hair, nails, or smooth skin. Reward systems often seem quite easy to develop and manage. Many parents assume a system will be simple, or determine ahead of time that a reward system will not work because they have tried and failed when using them in the past. Parents need assistance in understanding the mechanics, reasoning, and management of reward systems. A reward system that is created well, monitored daily, evaluated weekly, and altered frequently can be quite instrumental to the success of the entire behavior change program.

EMPHASIZING RELAPSE PREVENTION IN THE TREATMENT OF BODY-FOCUSED REPETITIVE BEHAVIORS

Because hair pulling and skin picking are relatively high-relapse behaviors, it is helpful to weave relapse prevention into the fabric of treatment. From the beginning of treatment (often in the first session), talk to parents about behavior change as a *process*. Again, using the example of weight loss can be useful. If a person goes on a diet and exercise program and loses 40 pounds, is he or she done? Does the person go back to eating whatever he or she wants and not exercising? If the person does, what will happen? The therapist will need to help parents and children to understand that the long-term maintenance of treatment gains depends on daily work over extended periods of time. The therapist should explain that as the months and years go by, strategies will be modified and will eventually become a way of life, not cumbersome "interventions." Another important point to make early on in treatment is that slips are normal and to be expected. It is all too common for parents (and sometimes therapists as well) to panic when a child who has been doing well with the BFRB has a setback and pulls or picks. It is important not only to expect these slips, but to predict them. Slips are normal and can illustrate what is working and, more importantly, what is not working with regard to treatment. The family will need help in order to treat slips as very informative occurrences. Slips are wonderful opportunities to problem-solve with a child and the parents as to why the slip happened. Both child and parents can then move forward armed with the knowledge of what to do when the same or similar circumstances arise in the future.

If slips are perceived as failures, both parents and children alike can then become distraught. In many cases, intense emotional reactions to slips can cause a relapse to occur. The therapist should educate clients and parents about the utility of slips and how to prevent relapse. It is the therapist's job to help families to navigate slips in a manner that addresses the parent's and child's emotional reactions and enables them to communicate clearly and problem-solve creatively through each different situation.

WORKING WITH COUPLES IN THE TREATMENT OF BODY-FOCUSED REPETITIVE BEHAVIORS IN ADULTS

This chapter has focused primarily on helping primary caretakers to assist a child or young adult to cope with a BFRB. Often, spouses need support as well. Most of the information included in this chapter (education, erroneous beliefs, common mistakes, and avoiding relapse) is relevant to helping a couple cope with a BFRB in the context of their marriage. Of greatest importance is to help the spouse to accept his or her loved one in a nonjudgmental, loving, nurturing way. Part of therapy may be focused on helping the person with a BFRB talk to his or her spouse about which behaviors or comments are helpful and which are not. The spouse may need some added support in order to provide the kind of loving help that may be required. Spouses, like parents, can feel as though they have a "solution" for their partner's problem but the partner "won't listen." Spouses often need special focus from the therapist to allow time for expressing their own feelings, frustrations, and fears. In addition, the therapist should teach spouses to listen to and respect their loved one's choices. Patients may wish to receive no help at all from their spouses or may desire a fair amount. Either way, both client and spouse need to develop clear communication skills that allow the client to express his or her needs and to know that his or her wishes will be respected.

CONCLUSION

When a child of any age enters therapy for a BFRB, the primary caregivers are going to need some therapy as well. Parents often present with misinformation, guilt, frustration, and tremendous anxiety regarding their child's behavior and ultimately their child's future. In addition, tension may be present as a result of conflict and/or control issues, resulting in deteriorating relationships between one or both parents and the child experiencing the BFRB.

The first step in treatment is to educate the family about the prevalence, etiology, course, and treatment of BFRBs. It is most helpful, at this stage, to instill hope about the treatment of these disorders and about their child's future. Treatment providers should expect that parents will have some complex and often intense feelings regarding the behavior. These feelings can be rooted in mistaken beliefs, patterns of maladaptive responses to the BFRB, or a parent's personal history with a problem. The therapist should encourage parents to express their feelings, fears, and frustrations while reassuring them that they are not alone, these feelings are common, and BFRBs do not simply affect the individual but have a far-reaching impact on the family.

Early in treatment, the therapist should validate parents' feelings of frustration and their impulses to "control" their child's behavior. Parents should be educated about common responses to BFRBs, including impatience, blaming, policing, and too much focus. Although these feelings and reactions are predictable and understandable, they certainly do not lead to behavior change for the child and ultimately can lead to shame, humiliation, and suffering for both parent and child.

During this phase of treatment, the therapist helps the family gain a different perspective regarding BFRBs and develop the skills necessary to effectively manage difficult emotions. The first step is to adopt patience, rather than impatience, thus fostering empathy and compassion for the child who is struggling to manage his or her behavior. Rather than blaming the child for the behavior, parents must learn to accept that with BFRBs there likely was a biological predisposition that set the stage for the pulling or picking. Instead of policing the behavior, parents are taught to relinquish control so that their child can accept some responsibility for the behavior and ultimately make steps toward change. Finally, parents are encouraged to focus on other aspects of their child, preferably what the child is good at, rather than what the child is currently struggling with. These changes are often difficult for parents to make and may require therapeutic support and guidance.

Attending to parents' feelings is not just a good idea—it is crucial for the successful treatment of a child with a BFRB. Although parents cannot control their child's pulling or picking behavior, they can control the atmosphere in the household. Therapy can help parents to establish a household atmosphere of openness and acceptance rather than helplessness, judgment, and blame. This shift alone will ease pressure and can sometimes serve to reduce a BFRB. The goal for treatment will then become to preserve the self-esteem and healthy development of their child, not simply to change the child's behavior. It is the therapist's job to keep this goal in focus and to redirect parents back to this goal when they become fearful and mistakenly focused on immediate change. Just as parents can become overly focused on "stopping the BFRB," the therapist can fall into this same trap. The focus of therapy should be kept on the child as a complex individual who is simply trying to get his or her needs met (and who has found a very effective way to do this). For successful treatment, the therapist will need to help both parents and child to understand what needs are being met by the BFRB and teach alternate ways to satisfy these needs.

Therapy is a process, and there will likely be slips along the way. Encourage families to appreciate slips because they allow for opportunities to demonstrate and practice new skills. These skills include better and clearer communication regarding the BFRB behavior, appropriate management of emotions such as disappointment, and the ability to effectively and creatively problem-solve future events. All of this is done with respect, validation of feelings, and acceptance of the BFRB as a small part of who the child is, not a summary of his or her identity. If these goals are kept in focus, therapy will be successful in terms of reduced BFRB behaviors, increased self-efficacy of the child, improved family dynamics, and renewed feelings of hope for the future.

REFERENCES

Franklin ME, Flessner CA, Woods DW, et al: The Child and Adolescent Trichotillomania Impact Project: descriptive psychopathology, functional impairment, comorbidity, and treatment utilization. J Dev Behav Pediatr 29:493–500, 2008

Mansueto CS, Golomb RG, Thomas AM, et al: A comprehensive model for behavioral treatment of trichotillomania. Cogn Behav Pract 6:23–43, 1999

Mouton-Odum S, Golomb R: Stay Out of My Hair! Parenting Your Child With Trichotillomania. Olney, MD, Goldum Publishing, 2009

INDEX

Page numbers printed in **boldface** *type refer to tables or figures.*